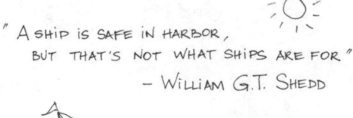

" A SHIP IS SAFE IN HARBOR,
   BUT THAT'S NOT WHAT SHIPS ARE FOR "
              — WILLIAM G.T. SHEDD

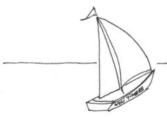

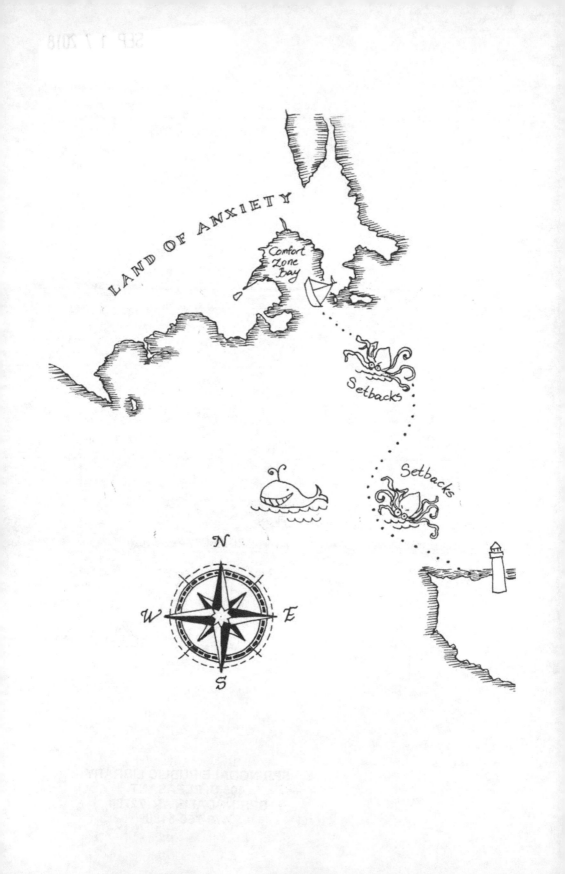

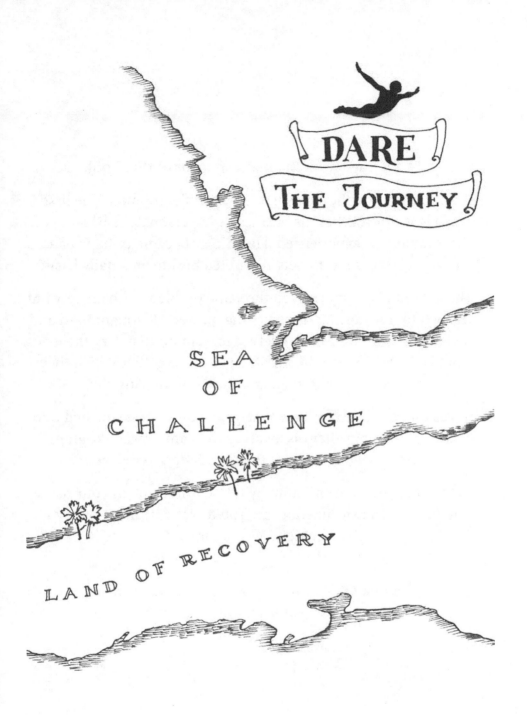

DARE
THE JOURNEY

SEA
OF
CHALLENGE

LAND OF RECOVERY

A message from the main sponsor of this Book

Let me tell you the story of two very different men. The first man lost control over his business and personal life because of the anxiety he experienced. He quickly became unhappy and unsuccessful as the anxiety disrupted his life on a daily basis.

The second man experienced the same problem with anxiety but learned to transform it into personal power. He fought hard and eventually won over his anxiety. He went on to marry the love of his life and built a dream life for them together which they now share with their son (and dog) in Austria.

I was that first man for four long years. I then transformed into the second man after discovering the Panic Away Program. Barry's work gave me the foundation to recover.

Let me tell you here and now, by taking this book in your hands you too can transform your life. You too can triumph over your anxiety. If you dare...

Szilard Koos
Future IT Solutions -Design and Development
(www.fitsolutions.at)

PRAISE FOR PANIC AWAY

"Funny; you know, of all the 'medical professionals' that I have been to over the years, alternate and mainstream, not one of them suggested your approach to the problem, yet it is so simple!"

"I never understood anxiety until it hit me 24/7. It was horrifying beyond words. I learned, through the program and the support of the wonderful people in your network, how to work through the anxiety. Not only have I learned to be me again, I have learned to take on wonderful challenges in my life and take chances toward a new life. I have moved to Florida, taken on a new job, and am now pursuing something I have always wanted to do. I would have never taken chances before anxiety. ... I stayed right in my little comfort zone. Words of thanks are not enough!"

"I honestly never thought I would be able to overcome my fears and anxieties; they had clouded my existence for so long. But the last two years have been unbelievable. I am now able to live my life to the full; every morning is like a new beginning. Every day seems so precious and I am making sure I do not miss one minute of it. I am 75 on Wednesday ... shshsh ... but I feel about 50 now that I am able to do all the things I have always dreaded doing. See what you've done, my husband can hardly keep up with me these days ... it's great!"

"I have suffered with panic attacks for 15 years and all the counseling, medication and books I have purchased within the 15 years just masked the fear, but never eliminated it for good. Your book was amazing from the first page to the last. Your knowledge has put me at peace and your wording was clear and understanding. Perfect."

"I am in tears (of joy) as I write this. I feel that I am no longer living in a mental prison. Yesterday, and today, I drove my car in traffic; traffic was my biggest fear, other than crowded places, and I did not panic. I am so happy about this."

"I feel pretty strongly about this book and what it has done for me after years and years of trying all sorts of different things from hypnotherapy to meditation to sheer 'mind-over-matter.' No more days and nights consumed by thoughts of panic attacks—it's just bliss. I love it."

"I cannot believe what an impact your program has made on my life. I have lived with OCD since I was in junior high and have had severe general anxiety my whole life. Your program has given me so much. I cannot believe how quickly it worked."

"Before taking your course I was drowned in general anxiety and panic attacks every time I left my house to the point that I never wanted to leave home. Now I am a happier person, a much better mom and my surroundings have changed incredibly. I never want to stay home and I will never send someone else to the grocery store again."

"I've suffered from GAD and claustrophobia for 18 years. I was using drugs and alcohol to get through flights. I felt very skeptical using this program at first but today I no longer need crutches to fly and no longer fear holidays! It has changed my life."

"I would drive around, anxious of what might happen. I was scared to go to work, and I was prohibiting myself from enjoying the outgoing life that I had once had. That has all changed; the daytime anxious feelings are now extremely rare, and panic is no longer a terror for me. Thank you for showing me the natural way out."

"My nervous system was shot after 33 years of alcohol & drugs. My psychiatrist (after telling me there was nothing wrong with me and I wasn't going mad), handed me a piece of paper with Panic Away scribbled on it. I went online immediately and ordered it. Long story short, it worked. Immediate results. Hope restored, journey continuing. Who would have thought God would use an Irishman to help me."

"A single panic attack I had at work one day stemmed into constant anxiety and body pains that I could not shake, until I received the help I needed from Barry McDonagh. As I write this, I find it so hard to believe I suffered from general anxiety the way I did. I'm doing things now that six years ago I would either have to really push myself to do, or I just wouldn't do at all. Simple pleasures like driving a car, going on vacation, speaking in front of a large group, going to New York City, or just simply talking one on one with a girl on a date."

"I have suffered from anxiety/panic disorder since I was 8 years old. I was diagnosed when I was in my mid to late 30s. My anxiety was making me a prisoner in my own home. I felt like I could not go out and do things because, 'What if I have a panic attack?' I'm now able to go out and do things with my husband that I never would have dreamed of doing a few years ago. I'm off of my anxiety medication and I feel wonderful. You were the one that put me on the path that I'm on now, and I thank you so much for it!"

"It's been 6 years now and your Panic Away program has been such a changing force in my life! My anxiety/panic was getting so bad that I had to quit my job that I loved! Thanks to you and your program, I have learned to work through my anxiety … and not let it overtake me ever again! My husband was there with me and learned the program too, to help me if I ever need a nudge :) We have helped so many people over the years who have anxiety/panic pointing them to your program. It works. Thank you from all of us!"

"I suffered from anxiety and panic attacks for 36 years. I had my first on the day of my eldest son's 2nd birthday party. It hit like a bolt out of the blue. I thought I was dying. I missed a lot of my children's activities. I had excuses for everything. Every time I was asked to a function I made up excuses as to why I couldn't go. Finally I found Panic Away some years ago. My life has since changed dramatically. I went to my son's wedding and started going out again. Not white knuckling it but really enjoying myself. I had my own business for a time, secured a high paying job with the Government and attended university. I am very grateful to have my life back and cannot thank Barry enough."

Official Sponsors of this Book

ACKNOWLEDGEMENTS

Much of this book is based on the way I healed my own anxiety disorder, but a great deal also comes from the many people I have had the good fortune of coaching over the years.

I have incorporated so much of their wisdom and insight into this new book that I really see it as collective effort rather than *my* book. I owe special thanks to Michelle Cavanaugh who has run my coaching program for the past several years. She has a unique way of explaining complex psychological topics so that everyone can grasp them quickly. She also suggested using the acronym DARE. I also want to thank everyone who has participated on my forum and in the group calls that I run. Their openness, insight, and eventual healing has inspired me to keep spreading the word that all anxiety can be healed no matter how long a person has been suffering.

I want to thank my developmental editor Stuart Horwitz, my copy editor Sharon Honeycutt as well as Shane Nestor for his encouragement to bring more fun and personal stories into the writing. Thank you Dr. Jay Polmar for the layout design and Yevgenia Watts for her unique artwork. I'd also like to thank Dr. Joan Swart,

PsyD for her research on the empirical evidence behind The DARE Response.

A big thank you to the following people for giving me insightful feedback during the writing process: Michelle Cavanaugh, Patrick Touhey, Padraig McCarthy, Ian Fergie, Elise Monte, Sue Booth, William Fernandez, Cameron Fancourt, Sarah Anderson, Alan Brady, Gil Yoh, and Alessandro Maltese. Lastly to my wife and family for their patience as I wrote this. Their support makes it possible. Thank you everyone for everything.

CONTENTS

PREFACE

There is nothing worse than wanting to run away and escape your own self. When you want to escape your own mind and body, it feels like there's nowhere to run. I know how that feels. I've been there.

I also know that right now you might feel like a small boat facing into a storm of anxiety and that just trying to concentrate on reading this book is an enormous challenge.

The first thing you must know is that it's going to be okay! You're going to get through this. In fact, not only are you going to get through this, but with the help of this book, you can journey to a place of full recovery and become a stronger person because of it. Anxiety is not a life sentence. It *is* absolutely curable.

A new era is dawning for people who suffer from anxiety, and this book is part of that movement. I'm going to share a truly transformative way to heal anxiety. This approach, called "The DARE Response," came about as a result of my own personal experience with healing anxiety. Its roots are in the new wave of positive psychology and the mindfulness movement that have become so popular in the last five to ten years. It's an approach that seeks to do away with the old model of simply managing and coping with anxiety; it seeks instead to heal the problem for good.

No matter how trapped and distraught you feel right now, this process can really work miracles for you as long as you commit to it. Your perseverance will navigate you through this storm and ensure you reach full recovery.

I'm not saying this journey is for everyone. I'm also not saying this will be easy. What I am saying is that if you stay the course, the rewards will be worth it. Together we'll fight to win back your peace of mind, your strength of will, and your joy in life.

INTRODUCTION

dare : v.

To confront boldly;
brave.

Anxiety is unpleasant. It often feels as if you're separated from ordinary life by a pane of glass. The doubt and confusion it causes are the hardest to deal with:

"Why is this happening to me?"

"Am I going mad?"

"Is my brain damaged?"

"Will this last forever?"

An anxiety disorder is difficult to understand unless you've experienced it firsthand. An anxiety disorder is not the kind of garden-variety stress everyone loves to talk about.

You hear people remark, "Yeah, I'm so stressed too" and "Hey, who isn't anxious—why are you complaining?" There's a *big* difference between anxiety and that kind of stress, and most people don't understand how all-consuming anxiety can be. They have no idea how terrifying a panic attack can feel or how uncomfortable a sensation like unreality can be. Your doctor may have a sympathetic ear, but unless they have experienced anxiety, they may never really 'get' what you are going through.

People who don't understand can often lose patience. They might say things like, "Come on, pull yourself together!" or "Just snap out of it!"

You try to explain to your very best friend that you can't make the wedding, and they think you're being selfish or you're not thinking of them on their big day. Your buddies want to go on a short hike, but you know that it's *way* too far out of your safe zone. They don't understand that you feel so shaken by anxiety that it's hard enough to think about leaving your house, not to mention having to walk in the wilderness, miles from a hospital.

In these situations, you want your companions to understand you're not avoiding them, but unfortunately, that's how it comes across. You need someone to understand how scary this damn thing feels, someone who can reassure you that you're not losing your mind.

It can be very hard to admit you have anxiety. How do you share with someone that sometimes you feel so out of control? That sometimes your mind fills with bizarre and shocking thoughts. You worry that if anyone knew what was going on in your head, they would call to have you locked up and your kids sent to a foster home.

So you make another excuse to get out of a social engagement, and in the meantime your sense of self-worth really takes a thrashing. You beat yourself up over it constantly:

> *"I mean really ... what the* heck *is wrong with me?! Why can't I just get up in the morning and not obsess about this anxiety and the day ahead? I used to be so carefree, and now I worry about having to sit still while getting my hair cut!"*

I'm not going to go on about this. You already know exactly how it feels. I mention it just to point out that it's perfectly normal to feel this way. You're not alone. You're not "losing it," and you don't have a serious health problem. Anxiety can play tricks on your mind. Of course, if you do have a health concern, _please_ make sure you get all the necessary examinations so that you can rule out those conditions.

But chances are excellent you're "simply" suffering from anxiety. I know you wish the doctor would just find some subtropical disease to explain all these sensations. At least then you could go about treating this or that disease.

If, on the other hand, you've been diagnosed with anxiety, then in all likelihood that really is what it is. Trust that diagnosis and don't second-guess it, fearing it might be something much worse.

You feel the way you do because of high levels of stress hormones in your system. We'll go through this in more detail later in this book, but basically our body's fight-or-flight response has gone a bit trigger-happy and is wreaking mental and emotional havoc.

YOU ARE NOT ALONE IN THIS

I know you might think your anxiety is very unique and singular to you, but I'm sorry to burst your bubble. It isn't. It's not one bit unique at all. In fact, it's as boring, ordinary, and common as everyone else's anxiety.

There are literally millions of perfectly sane, normal people who have the exact same problem you do. (In the United States alone, approximately 40 million American adults aged eighteen and older are estimated to have an anxiety disorder.) _So if you suffer from anxiety, you're actually quite normal._

No matter how deranged and shocking your anxious thoughts are, I guarantee you there's someone close to you who is also suffering in silence. No matter how bad your panic attacks are, there are millions of people that experience them in the exact same manner—with the exact same unusual sensations—as you. Millions of perfectly sane people suffer in silence because stress hormones cause an oversensitized nervous system.

"BUT I FEEL LIKE I'M LOSING IT!"

You're not going nuts. If you could flick a magic switch that caused an immediate reduction of all the stress hormones floating through your bloodstream, you would suddenly feel a whole lot more normal again. The sense of unreality would end and so would the tornado of anxious thoughts tearing through your mind.

Have you ever heard the saying, if you think you're going nuts, you probably aren't? One of the goals of this book is to assure you that you're perfectly okay and that you can indeed end your anxiety problem.

The fact is anxiety is incredibly treatable, but very few people tell you that! I've been teaching people how to end anxiety issues for over ten years, and I can't stress enough that this problem is entirely curable. All it takes is the *right* guidance and your commitment to get better. This book outlines exactly how you can end your anxiety problem and move toward a greater sense of personal freedom. Getting you back to your old, carefree self again is the goal.

Let me briefly explain how it happened for me. My anxiety problem started with a panic attack. If you've experienced panic attacks, I bet you remember your first. Mine was on a Sunday afternoon in a church in Dublin. I was eighteen years old and had been out celebrating my final school exams the night before.

I was desperately hung over, sitting a few deep in the church pew, when a series of really intense bodily sensations suddenly overcame me. My heart was pounding through my chest. I couldn't catch my breath, and pins and needles started to spread down the side of my chest and arms. It was the most alarming series of bodily sensations I had ever experienced.

My first thought was, "What if I'm having a heart attack?" As soon as I had that thought, my anxiety spiked into a state of panic! The fear I felt was like an electrical shock to my stomach.

I needed to get outside, so I excused myself and rushed toward the exit at the back of the church. Standing outside, the physical sensations lessened slightly, and I thought the worst had passed. Then another wave of panic and fear hit me even harder.

I wanted desperately to ask someone for help, but what would I say to them? I looked for a friendly face, but no one made eye contact. Would asking for help just make me feel more helpless and afraid? Would they even know what to do? I paced up and down, thinking about how far I was from the nearest hospital, when I felt the sensations lessen slightly. I decided to try to make it home. I got my bike and walked it slowly back home, carefully trying not to aggravate the sensations again.

When I eventually got home, I told no one and hid in my house for days. That was week one. What followed were about 500 more days of really high general anxiety as well as additional panic attacks. I went from being a young man who could travel the world with ease to someone who became afraid to leave his house. During that period of time, I experienced just about every anxious sensation possible. It was like a crash course in anxiety disorders. You name it, I felt it, from strange bodily sensations to intrusive thoughts and depersonalization.

The turning point came one evening. I remember it clearly. I had really hit rock bottom and was lying on the floor of my bedroom, wishing the anxiety would end, when this flash of insight came to me. It was like seeing my thought processes from a distance. For the first time, I could clearly see how I had been approaching this all *wrong*. I was fueling my anxiety problem by the way I was responding to each and every anxious thought that crossed my mind.

That one insight eventually led to the end of my panic attacks and constant anxiety! It was like a complete *retooling* of my thought process related to anxiety from a wrong way, to a daring, new way. The illusion of fear that the anxiety held me under was shattered, and from that point forward I started to win back my freedom.

I wanted to share that insight with others, so I eventually wrote it all down and posted it online. The response was almost immediate. People told me they were making massive improvements in their anxiety from the insights I shared. Now I had validation that this same approach could work for other people too. From there I wrote my first book, *Panic Away*, which later went on to become an international best seller. That was ten years ago, and since then I have had the privilege of coaching people from every walk of life. I have taught CEOs and soccer moms, famous celebrities and military personnel.

What makes my approach unique is the speed of recovery that people achieve. The lessons and insights I share are simple and get results fast. For example:

- People who could not leave their homes are now flying on holidays overseas.

- People who could not drive to the end of their roads are now driving across the country.

- TV presenters and entertainers who were about to quit their jobs are now doing their best work yet.

- Mothers and fathers who could not attend their kids' school plays are now participating fully in their children's lives.

You name it, if anxiety is the problem, I've seen it and helped someone somewhere overcome it. It has been a privilege to be able to play a part in thousands of people's recovery from anxiety. Helping them get their life back after years of unnecessary anxiety and fear is rewarding work. Over the course of the past decade, the route to healing anxiety for good became clearer and clearer to me and motivated me to write this book you're holding.

In this book, you'll discover how to:

- put an end to anxious and intrusive thoughts

- stop the occurrence of panic attacks and end general anxiety

- face any anxious situation you've been avoiding—driving, shopping, flying, socializing, etc.

- regain your confidence and feel like your old self again, no matter how long you've been suffering

The insights I'll share with you really can undo years of anxiety—and here's what truly sets this book apart: You'll not only learn how to end your anxiety problem, but you'll also *discover how to turn this problem into a personal triumph.* You'll have the opportunity to discover the meaning in this struggle and develop a new hidden strength within yourself.

People who eventually find me usually do so after they've gone through a wide range of therapies and treatments, everything from alternative therapies to the more traditional route of anti-anxiety medications. I'm sure you've tried an exhaustive list of things already. Because we lead complicated lives, we often expect the solutions to our problems to be expensive and complicated too. In fact, we trust expensive, complicated solutions over simple ones, even when most approaches overcomplicate recovery. The approach I teach, called The DARE Response, does the opposite for you. It simplifies recovery.

The reason that many of these other approaches fail is that they're based on an old model of "anxiety management." The culture of anxiety management is so pervasive in today's society that medication and distraction techniques are the only solutions people know. Managing anxiety, however, is not a real long-term solution. The name itself gives you a clue to its impact: you learn to manage anxiety but not to heal it. You might get temporary relief, but the anxiety inevitably returns, and you haven't developed the confidence to deal with it.

I don't teach anxiety management. I teach people how to heal their anxiety *so they can get back to living their life again to its fullest.*

Anxiety causes you to become stuck in a stagnant state of fear. Learning how to skillfully move with the anxious discomfort that you feel removes you from that state of fear. Moving *with* anxiety places you back into a state of flow, which eventually frees you from an anxious state. The DARE Response teaches you that simple movement.

The unusual thing about The DARE Response is that it's not designed to get rid of your anxiety; it's designed to *get rid of your fear of the anxiety.* It's your resistance to and struggle with anxiety that keeps you trapped. A bit like quicksand, the more you struggle, the deeper you sink. When you employ The DARE Response, your anxious mind is taken out of the way, allowing your nervous system to desensitize.

I'm not suggesting that once you master this approach you'll never experience anxiety again. That's unrealistic. Life has its challenges that will cause anxiety to rise up again at times just like it does for me. The difference, however, is that you won't get trapped in that anxious state any longer. Instead, you'll pass through it with ease.

Although the insights I had during my own recovery were unique to me, I don't for a moment claim to be the originator of this new approach. I call it the "new approach" for healing anxiety because up until just a few short years ago, almost every therapeutic treatment for anxiety was based on that old model of managing the problem indefinitely. Thankfully in recent years, a quiet revolution has been happening in psychology, and now we're starting to see new therapies emerge that truly address anxiety and heal it at its core. Some examples of these therapies include mindfulness-based cognitive therapy (MBCT) and acceptance and commitment therapy (ACT).

It's not that these new psychological approaches were just developed. In fact, many great doctors and psychiatrists in the 1950s and 1960s, such as the late Drs. Viktor Frankl and Claire Weekes, advocated tirelessly for them as the only truly effective treatments for anxiety. Unfortunately back then, the dominant thinking was that anxiety was a permanent condition that had to be managed or medicated away.

I believe over the next ten years this new approach will become the mainstream therapeutic approach for healing all anxiety because of the efficiency of results it achieves and the speed at which those results occur. My contribution is to help make this approach as simple and easy to apply as possible. (You can read all about the hard science behind The DARE Response in the appendix of this book.)

You see, when people are anxious or in the grip of a panic attack, they need really simple and clear instructions. The DARE Response is simple if nothing else. It's an approach that can be applied to all manifestations of anxiety be it general anxiety, panic attacks, OCD or social anxiety.

"You can only take people as far as you have gone" **Old English Proverb**

Often times the best insights and breakthroughs can come from outside the world of academia. While I have graduated in psychology, I am not a clinical psychologist, therapist or doctor. My unique understanding and skill in this area comes from direct personal experience of ending my own anxiety. What I feel makes me more than qualified to help you is my ten-year track record of helping countless people end their anxiety disorders.

Before we get into the details of The DARE Response, I would like you to think of this book as a journey we're taking together. I'm going to be asking you to leave the safe haven of your comfort zone and travel with me to full recovery. This won't always be an easy journey. There will be times when you'll feel like quitting, but please don't. I know you have what it takes to get there.

YOU'RE HERE BECAUSE YOU'RE READY

You've been dealing with this as bravely as you can, and all you need now is someone to help you navigate your way to recovery.

You wouldn't be reading this book if you didn't have what it takes to get there. I know sometimes you've felt like giving up, but you didn't. You kept searching. I salute your courage and thank you for placing your trust in me. These are not just words on a page. I'm here rooting for you.

All the suffering in silence that you've endured, all the emotional pain—none of it has been in vain. It's served a greater purpose in your life. You're reading this book because you're now ready for this bold journey.

Let's be clear about one thing: This is the fastest approach I know to permanently heal your anxiety, but your anxiety symptoms won't vanish in a day. What you'll feel instead is a shift. It's a bit like turning down the volume on an irritating radio that's broadcasting static. You'll be able to go for longer and longer periods of time without even noticing this radio. Eventually you'll have to strain your ears to hear it. And then ... silence!

"HOW WILL I KNOW WHEN I'VE REACHED A FULL RECOVERY?"

You're very near a full recovery when you're no longer concerned with whether your anxious sensations are present or not. Note, I'm not saying "when you no longer feel anxious sensations." That will come later. The most crucial point to reach right now is to *get comfortable with your anxious discomfort.*

After that, things get a lot easier. You'll notice that you can go long periods of time without thinking about anxiety. You stop "checking in" all the time to see how you're feeling until eventually you feel much less anxious in general. The anxiety may pop back up from time to time to pay you a visit, but you no longer fear it because you have the skill set to move through it quickly again.

Before we begin, I want you to take a moment right now and imagine what your life will be like without your anxiety issue.

What will that mean for you? Maybe it will mean sharing more fun experiences with friends and family. Maybe it will mean traveling to a new country or visiting friends far away. Maybe it will simply mean being able to do everyday things like drive, shop, and move about without the oppressive feeling of being anxious all the time. Whatever it is, I want you to think about what that will look like for you. We'll come back to this exercise at the end of the book.

Now, let's begin your journey to full recovery. There really is a light at the end of the tunnel. (And *NO, it's not a train coming at you!*)

This book is accompanied by a free app for your smartphone or desktop. Please go now to www.DareResponse.com/app and download the app so that you can access audios to help you recovery faster.

YOU'RE THE CURE

The very first thing to be aware of as we set off on this journey is that it's *okay not to feel okay*. That's the launching point. All the months or years that anxiety has been with you can really take their toll. It may have been a very long time since you really felt like yourself.

A person who experiences frequent panic attacks or general anxiety is constantly bombarded with a cocktail of stress hormones. This bombardment not only makes your nervous system highly sensitized to stress, but it also leaves you feeling eerily cut off from the world. Reality may have gone a bit weird, but that's okay. Now that you know the anxiety you feel is simply due to your body's stress response, you can begin to feel more and more comfortable about it.

The second thing to be aware of is that *you are not a weak or cowardly person for having an anxiety problem.* I have worked with some of the bravest people you could ever hope to meet. Police officers, firefighters and military personnel who could perform incredibly brave feats in the line of duty and yet who were tormented by anxiety issues while off duty. I once worked with a Police Chief – a decorated officer who supervises over 300 police officers – who couldn't sit in the barbers for a haircut. He dealt with highly pressurized situations every working day and felt very much in control, yet in the barber's chair he felt out of control as he had a panic attack there once before. So don't think of yourself as being weak or less courageous than others just because you suffer from anxiety. Far from it.

I assure you that the anxiety you feel is not that different from the anxiety experienced by all the other people who have successfully used this approach. Over the years I have come across such a wide range of anxiety issues that nothing surprises me anymore. Panic disorder, generalized anxiety disorder, social anxiety, OCD, Pure O: behind all the different manifestations is the same thing—anxiety.

I don't like to subcategorize anxiety into individual labels or even call it a "disorder." I mentioned those terms above only so that you're clear that what I'm talking about is what you've heard. Labels are useful only for defining an experience a person is going through right at that time in life. They should not be understood as something that now makes up a person's personality or as something they will have forever.

People tend to overidentify with clinical labels once they have been given one by their doctor or mental health professional. Yet an anxiety disorder is simply an experience that a person moves through, just like a period of grief or sadness. Would we give a person with a broken heart or someone suffering from grief a label for life? No, yet people who go through a period of anxiety sometimes end up believing that this diagnosis, this label, is now a part of who they are.

"HOW FAST WILL I BE ABLE TO END MY ANXIETY PROBLEM?"

The speed and manner in which each individual heals their anxiety is always different, so it's impossible to say exactly how fast and in what way it will happen for you. In general, however, it unfolds in stages for most people. Before I explain what those stages look like, I want to share an important point: *The speed of your recovery is determined by your willingness to experience your anxiety in the right way.* Up until now you've been experiencing anxiety in the wrong way. I'm going to teach you how to experience it in the right way, and paradoxically by doing this, you can heal it quickly. It's a bit like turning a release valve the wrong way and just closing it tighter. You need to turn it in a counterintuitive manner to cause a release.

Once you apply this new approach, you'll move through some predictable stages:

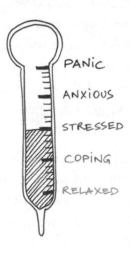

Stage 1. First of all, if panic attacks are a problem for you, they become less frequent in a very short space of time. This happens because you learn how to remove the fear of the bodily sensations that have been triggering them. Your confidence in your body's ability to handle the stress starts to return, enabling you to visit again the places you may have been avoiding.

Stage 2. Next, your level of general anxiety starts to go down from, say, an 8 out of 10 to a 4 or 5. This stage of reducing general anxiety is a slower process as you have to allow time for your nervous system to become less sensitized. This healing process is not linear; it's not like the mending of a broken bone. You'll likely move forward and then back and then leap forward again.

Stage 3. As your general anxiety decreases, anxious thoughts or worries appear less frequently. This happens because your fearful response to them has reduced. If they felt like a punch to the stomach before, now they might feel just like a mild annoyance and not something that really shocks you anymore. It's also at this stage that uncomfortable feelings like derealization (feelings of unreality) start to diminish.

Stage 4. This is a transition phase where you move from always feeling anxious to noticing the absence of the anxiety. If anxiety has been present for many years, this stage in the process can feel strange, like a storm that's been raging for so long that suddenly goes quiet. "Can it really be gone?" you ask yourself. "What if it comes back worse than ever?" Returning to the metaphor we used earlier, this stage can feel a bit like being freed from prison ... where you're still worrying that you might get thrown back in at any moment.

Stage 5. Next comes a setback! Yes, sorry, but they will come. Setbacks can be a major blow to your newfound confidence. You thought you were free of anxiety, and now it seems to be back and as bad as ever. You think to yourself: "I knew it would come back. I'll never be rid of this! There *is* something seriously wrong with me after all." Many people flounder here because they get so upset and frustrated. This is a normal response, but it's essential at this point to understand that setbacks are part of the recovery. Don't give up; you're so very close to the finish. This is a crucial phase you must pass through, a bit like a final test to see if you're really ready to let go of your anxiety. Remember, it's truly darkest before the dawn.

Stage 6. Finally, after some more time practicing, you realize that it's been a few weeks since you gave much thought at all to anxiety. This is a sign that you're almost recovered from the "sensitization" of anxiety. Always bear in mind that setbacks can happen—sometimes even years later and without warning—but for the most part it's just a matter of staying the course from here on out and enjoying your newfound freedom.

The above stages are typical of how recovery happens for most people. As I mentioned, not everyone experiences the same pattern as anxiety manifests differently for each individual. You may deal only with anxious thoughts and not bodily sensations. Or maybe you have a problem not only with general anxiety but with panic attacks as well, which is why I added a special chapter on "The DARE Response for Panic Attacks."

I like to sometimes imagine the process of recovery described above like the sun coming out from behind a dark cloud and shining its light on a thick fog. The fog represents anxiety and how it traps you in a confused and fearful state. As you apply The DARE Response, the sun appears, and its warmth begins to lift the fog.

Sometimes the weather changes, and the fog rolls back in. The temperature drops, and the fear returns again. These are your setbacks. However, if you stay focused and practice The DARE Response, the sun reappears and lifts the fog once more.

The journey of recovery is done at each individual's own speed. Please don't compare yourself to others. There will always be people moving faster or slower than you toward recovery. Allow yourself to heal in your own time.

"WHY DO I HAVE THIS ANXIETY PROBLEM?"

I'm sure you've wondered several times why anxiety is a problem for you and not others—especially if it came totally out of the blue (e.g., panic attacks). Research indicates that there is a certain percentage of the population who have a genetic predisposition to anxiety. I believe most people I come across in my work fall into this category, this predisposition toward "anxiety sensitivity." If you're identified as having this genetic trait, it doesn't mean, however, that you'll develop a problem with anxiety. What it does mean is that you're more susceptible to feelings of anxious sensitizations than others.

For this group of people, the catalyst for the anxiety disorder to manifest is usually a trigger like extreme exhaustion (mental/emotional/physical) or sudden upheavals like a bereavement, illness, trauma, or the end of a relationship (separation). Sometimes anxiety doesn't spring from one particular life event. For these people, it originates because they haven't been looking after themselves properly (e.g., not eating right, not getting enough sleep, or consuming too much caffeine and alcohol). Poor diet and not getting the right amounts of key nutrients is a real trigger for many. There are other environmental factors that are known to make people more prone to developing an anxiety disorder. For example, losing someone early in childhood or overbearing or aggressive/domineering parenting can make some more prone to anxiety later in life.

Please be aware that if there is a specific identifiable cause for the anxiety, such as mental or physical abuse or other factors like addictions or clinical depression, then therapy is extremely important to help resolve that. But even when those issues have begun to be deeply dealt with, The DARE Response can be of great benefit, providing an immediate clarity of mind to remember all the work that's been done. The DARE Response offers an approach that makes it possible to address the anxiety in the here and now.

ANXIOUS CONTRACTIONS

Life is movement. It's dynamic and pulsating like a swift moving river. To be in a contented and happy state is to be in a state of flow where your thoughts and feelings follow a natural current and there is no inner friction or need to check in on your anxiety every five minutes. When you feel in flow, your body feels light and your mind becomes spontaneous and joyful.

Anxiety and fear are the total opposite.

They're the contractions of life. When we get scared, we contract in fear. Our bodies become stiff and our minds become fearful and rigid. If we hold that contracted state, we eventually cut ourselves off from life. We lose flexibility. We lose our flow.

We can think of this a bit like pulling a muscle. When a muscle is overused and tired, its cells run out of energy and fluid. This can lead to a sudden and forceful contraction, such as a cramp. This contraction is painful and scary as it comes without warning.

In the same way, we can be living our lives with a lot of stress and exhaustion, similar to holding a muscle in an unusual position for too long. If we fail to notice and take care of this situation, we can experience an intense and sudden moment of anxiety or even panic. I call this an "anxious contraction," and it can feel quite painful. Learning how to respond correctly to this anxious contraction is crucial and determines how quickly we release it.

Anxious contractions happen to almost everyone at some point in their lives. We suddenly feel overwhelmed with anxiety as our body experiences all manner of intense sensations, such as a pounding heart or a tight chest or a dizzy sensation. Our anxiety level then is maybe an 8 or 9 out of 10. We recoil in fear and spiral into a downward loop of more fear and anxiety. Some might say they had a spontaneous panic attack while others might describe the feeling as being very "on edge."

THE ANXIETY LOOP

It's at this point in time where people get split into those that develop an anxiety disorder and those that don't. The real deciding factor is whether a person gets caught in the "anxiety loop" or not. The anxiety loop is a mental trap, a vicious cycle of fearing fear. Instead of ignoring anxious thoughts or bodily sensations, the person becomes acutely aware and paranoid of them.

"What if I lose control and do something crazy?"

"What if those sensations come back again while I'm in a meeting?"

"What if it's a sign of a serious health problem?"

This trap is akin to quicksand. Our immediate response is to struggle hard to free ourselves, but it's the wrong response. The more we struggle, the deeper we sink.

ANXIETY TRAP

STRESSED

ANXIOUS

PANICKED

LIFE

Anxiety is such a simple but costly trap to fall into. All your additional worry and stress make the problem worse, fueling more anxiety and creating a vicious cycle or loop. It's like spilling gasoline onto a bonfire: the more you fear the bodily sensations, the more intense they feel. I've seen so many carefree people go from feeling fine one day to becoming fearful of everyday situations simply because they had one bad panic attack and then got stuck in this anxious loop of fearing fear. But there is great hope.

As strange as it sounds, the greatest obstacle to healing your anxiety is you. You're the cure. Your body wants to heal your anxiety as much as you do. All you need to learn is a new and better response—the kind of response that gets your anxious mind out of the way so that your nervous system can unwind and desensitize. You can do that with The DARE Response. This new response will enable you to step out of the anxiety loop and join with life again.

Before we continue, I want to compliment you on your commitment, having read this far into the book. Now stay with me as it's about to get interesting. In the following chapter I'm going to share The DARE Response with you. It's designed to end your problem for good, but I really need your full commitment from here on in. Your level of commitment determines how fast and effective your recovery will be.

THE DARE RESPONSE

Qui audet adipiscitur

Who dares wins

Anxiety is not a monster out to get you. I know it feels like that most of the time, but it isn't. I also know you fear it might kill you or drive you insane, but it won't.

You're safe. You have to trust that.

Your anxiety is not an attacker. It's an internal tug-of-war you're having with yourself. No monster is chasing you. Instead, this is your body's own misguided way of trying to protect you. It's trying to do what it thinks is best for you.

The tools you've been using up until now haven't been working, so you have to drop your old coping strategies and adopt a new approach. The DARE Response teaches you to have a radically new relationship with your anxiety. It teaches you to stop seeing your anxiety as an oppressive force but rather a neutral energy that can be channeled to your benefit.

It entails learning a new response to anxiety in order to become free of it. There are four simple steps:

Defuse
Allow
Run Toward
Engage

STEP 1. *DEFUSE*

Anxiety is nothing more than nervous energy in your body. This energy rises and falls just like waves on the ocean. Think of it as if you're bobbing around in the ocean and every now and then a wave rises up in front of you. These are the waves of nervous energy. When you resist the wave, it tosses you around and scares you, but when you move with it, you ride up and over it and eventually lose your fear of the waves.

The waves of anxiety rise up, peak, and then fall back down. They always peak and then subside away. Up and down they go. They become a problem (a disorder) only if you respond to them in the wrong way.

The first step of The DARE Response retrains how you immediately respond to anxiety. It's your first point of contact with the anxiety, and it's a very quick and easy step to implement.

Anxiety often comes from out of nowhere and then escalates really fast. As we saw in the previous chapter, anxiety's initial trigger can be caused by several different things (e.g., exhaustion, stress, poor diet), but it's rapidly escalating because you're going against the grain of your nervous arousal. You're responding to it the *wrong way.*

The biggest mistake most people make when anxiety strikes is to get caught up in "what if" thoughts.

What if my heart doesn't stop pounding?

What if I have a panic attack here in the car?

What if this constant anxiety doesn't go away?

What if I faint? Who will help me?

What if my mind never stops obsessing with these thoughts?

Since prehistoric times our minds have been wired to seek out potential threats and to then avoid them. The world we lived in then was often a life-or-death environment, and "what ifs" were a useful cognitive process that developed to keep us out of immediate danger.

What if that shadow behind that bush is a predator? Best to back away.

Today, however, it's rare (fortunately!) to encounter a life-or-death moment, so our minds turn inwards instead, looking for those same life-threatening situations that are almost always imagined or exaggerated.

What if that pounding heart means I'm about to have a heart attack?

What if I lose my job and can't feed myself or my family?

Notice that these "what ifs" almost never revolve around good things potentially happening, like:

What if someone surprises me with good news today?

What if the doctor says I'm in great health?

Our thoughts didn't evolve like this because, in prehistoric times, it was better to be cautious and guarded than optimistic and carefree.

If anxious "what ifs" aren't responded to correctly and quickly defused, they tend to spiral out of control, leaping from one catastrophic thought to another. Before you know it, these "what ifs" have triggered a tidal wave of adrenaline and fear.

What if? ... What if? ... And then what if?

You can't stop the initial waves of anxiety or the "what if" thoughts that cross your mind. They manifest outside your control. What you can always control is your response to them.

In order to defuse anxious "what ifs," you need to answer the question in the right way and limit the potential for the anxiety to increase.

A good response to a "what if" is: **"So what!"**

What if my heart doesn't stop pounding?

So what! My heart's an incredibly strong muscle. This is nothing more than a light workout for it.

What if I have a panic attack here in the car?

So what! I'll pull over and get through it like I've always done in the past.

What if I faint in public? Who will help me?

So what! If I faint, I faint. Someone will help me, and in two minutes I'll be conscious again.

What if my mind never stops obsessing with these thoughts?

So what! Thoughts are just thoughts and can't harm me. Eventually my anxious mind will settle, and the thoughts will dissipate.

It doesn't matter if you don't fully believe in your own responses to these questions. The key point here is to quickly defuse the buildup of fear by answering the "what ifs" in the right way with a strong "so what" attitude. Answering with **"so what"** is effective because it neutralizes the fear and places you back into a position of power.

If **"so what"** doesn't feel like the appropriate response for you, then come up with your own response like "whatever" or "oh well." Some members of my coaching program like to be less passive and more direct, so they jokingly say *WGAF* ("Who gives a f***!"). The important thing is to illicit a dismissive attitude toward your fears. As long as you come up with something dismissive of the initial "what if" thought, it will have the right effect.

Oftentimes there is no clear "what if" thought that you can identify, rather just a general feeling of foreboding that comes with the wave of anxious discomfort.

You can defuse that anxious foreboding of general anxiety quickly in the exact same manner by saying "**Whatever,** it's just nervous arousal, no big deal."

Defusing all anxiety with a strong attitude of **"so what" / "whatever"** is the first important step in The DARE Response. It quickly disarms the buildup of tension and gets you moving in the same direction as the nervous arousal instead of resisting it. It's a great start, but you now need to use the next step of the response to discharge the anxiety even further.

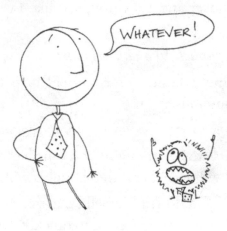

DEFUSE

STEP 2. *ALLOW IT*

Now that you've started to respond to anxiety in the right way, it's crucial you keep going by releasing all resistance so that any anxiety that's still present can dissipate even faster. You do this by *accepting the anxiety that you feel and allowing it to manifest in whatever way it wishes.*

You see, fear and anxiety can come on so suddenly that almost everyone's initial response to it is the same. We resist it. It's human nature to want to avoid an uncomfortable experience like anxiety. We'd rather run away from it or try to block it out. Unfortunately, no one has ever told us that's the wrong response to have. It's the wrong response because when we fight anxiety, that effort traps us with the same force we put into trying to fight it. When we run from it, it chases us with the same speed of our escape.

You'll always be stuck in a state of fear if you're always trying to keep your distance from it.

YOU CAN'T OUTRUN ANXIETY; YOU NEED TO MOVE WITH IT.

An anxiety disorder is exhausting because it's your own resistance repeatedly coming back at you. If you're feeling strong, sometimes you can fight off the anxious feelings for a while, but as soon as your guard comes down, it's back and as strong as ever. So how do you stop fighting it and move with it? You drop the resistance and embrace it. You allow it to be present. You can start to do that by repeating to yourself:

I accept and allow this anxious feeling.

I accept and allow this anxious feeling.

Allowing anxiety to be stops the mental friction and gives your nervous system an opportunity to wind down. Going back to our wave analogy, *allowing* enables you to gracefully move up and over the top of the wave.

So no matter what the bodily sensation or thought is that makes you anxious, you must learn to experience it in the right way. Allow it to be present, and then come to accept it for what it is—nervous arousal and nothing more. This wave of nervous arousal is happening. You may never find out why it's manifesting, but for right now that's not important. What is important is how you respond to it.

What we resist persists, and *what we accept, we can transform.* When we fully accept our anxiety by allowing it to be, without begrudging it, it then goes through a subtle transformation. As Lama Govinda said, "We are transformed by what we accept."

In essence, you must learn to get comfortable in your anxious discomfort.

Most of the things in life that we have to come to accept are not pleasant; they just are what they are. It's the same with nervous energy. The secret to recovery, however, is that once you reach a point where you really allow and accept it, it begins to fall away and discharge naturally. It's the paradox that is central to healing anxiety.

So from now on, I want you to stop asking yourself:

Will I feel okay today?

Instead, ask yourself:

What level of anxious discomfort am I willing to embrace today in order to heal?

Just like an athlete who embraces discomfort in order to achieve their end goal, you're embracing anxiety in order to get where you need to be.

Before I give you some examples of how to allow anxiety to be present, it's important to be aware that none of this is about giving in to your fears or anxiety. It's about having a new, almost detached relationship with it, a bit like a curious observer mindfully watching the waves of anxiety rise and fall. As you do that, you move more easily *with* your anxious discomfort rather than against it.

When you resist anxiety, you move against it, creating a further buildup of internal tension, making it unable to discharge. Don't turn away from anxiety; that never works. *Turn into it, allow it, and move with it.* When done correctly, this has a great healing effect on your nervous system, allowing it to desensitize from the anxious state you've been keeping it stuck in.

LET THE UNINVITED GUEST BE WELCOME

The reality is that healing anxiety is totally counterintuitive. You have to really move with it in order to be free of it. *"This is crazy,"* you might be thinking, *"to invite more crazy!"* But the fact is you have to accept and embrace your anxiety in order for it to leave.

Here's an example of how to allow the anxiety you feel. Say to yourself:

I'm no longer going to battle with you, anxiety. I call a truce. Come closer to me now, and sit down beside me. It's okay. I'm allowing you to stay. I accept and allow this anxious feeling. I accept and allow these anxious thoughts.

This open, warm invitation of accepting and allowing the anxious discomfort you feel to be with you is very freeing. Remove the resistance and allow your body to freely vibrate with all this nervous energy that you feel in your body. When done with real intention, you really flow with your nervous energy rather than rubbing with friction against it. You're declaring a truce between you and that which you've been fighting for so long. This is a really important moment and a turning point in your recovery.

"Attend and befriend your fear" as Tara Brach would say. Before, you resisted each and every sensation because your anxious mind thought that was the right thing to do, but now you're learning to sit with it in friendly curiosity, allowing it to be as it is without any desire to stop or control it.

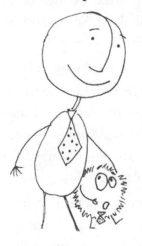

So every time you feel a wave of nervous energy, you can bob up and down with it as it rises and falls. Or you can treat it like a friend coming over to visit. Pretend you're actually glad to see it again. You're inviting it in so it can spend time with you.

Oh, look who's come to visit! Take a seat. I'm glad you showed up!"

ALLOW

Your anxiety won't escalate if you welcome it like this because you're moving with it without resistance or suppression. It will now naturally start to discharge.

Allow the anxiety to manifest in whatever way it wishes, physically or mentally. If it wants to make your throat feel tight, go ahead and let it. If it wants to make your heart pound, great. If it wants to make your mind race with wild thoughts, let it be your guest. Let your body vibrate with the nervous arousal without any hindrance so it can then start to unwind.

As you move with your nervous arousal, it may morph into different thoughts or sensations. As it does this, think to yourself:

That's interesting that you're now giving me this new sensation. Oh well ... whatever, *you're allowed.*

I accept and allow this anxious feeling. I accept and allow this anxious feeling.

Feel the rhythm of those words as they gently nudge you out of a stuck state and into a sense of flow with this nervous arousal.

I'm not suggesting this will be pleasant; of course it won't be. There's nothing pleasant or enjoyable about fear or anxiety, but unfortunately you really don't have a choice if you want it to dissipate naturally. You have to move along with it. Let this uninvited guest be welcome. Never get upset when anxiety shows up at your door. Smile and be the perfect host: invite it in, sit it down, and serve it tea.

If you're a visual type, give the anxiety a mental image like a ridiculous cartoon character. Come up with a great nickname for it. Imagine it about a foot tall, telling you about all the terrible things that might happen. Give your new friend a comical squeaky voice like it's just inhaled a can of helium. It bursts through your front door no bigger than a small dog squeaking profusely

Use whatever visual image for the anxiety that works for you. What's important is to bring your sense of humor into play and make it totally absurd. *Be open and playful with your anxiety.* You're not threatened by this cartoon character screaming red alert. You step back and just smile at its anxious rants. Get used to this cartoon character making dramatic entrances. It loves to show up at the most inopportune times! Once you're okay with that, you'll feel no anxious impact from it.

With a bit of practice, you can actually see the arrival of anxiety as a bit ridiculous. You can smile to yourself each time this character jumps on your shoulder or is in your ear, warning you about the next big threat that's about to befall you. The lighter you can make of the anxiety, the more allowing of it you'll become, and the faster you'll heal. Don't underestimate this open and playful attitude.

I know as you read this you may be feeling somewhat skeptical. That's natural. You fear that allowing anxiety into your life is only going to make it worse, right?

What if I allow it in and it gets worse? What if it all gets too much for me to handle?

Everyone has the same initial fear, but trust me: allowing anxiety to be works incredibly well. You won't get more anxious. In fact, the more welcoming you can be, the faster your anxiety level will drop. With continued practice, you'll discover this fact for yourself.

Your fear of what the anxiety might do to you is what has you stuck and trapped in anxiety. *It's your fear of fear that causes the whole problem.* When you decide to no longer play that game, you become free. You might think this approach sounds too simplistic to work. It couldn't possibly work for your complex anxiety problem, right?

I want you take a leap of faith and trust this simple approach. Trust me enough to at least try it for one week. Once you start to feel your anxiety reduce, you'll then have evidence to confirm that this is the right approach to take. Many great teachers have taught a very similar approach to healing fear and anxiety, but unfortunately those teachings have been drowned out by the more complex anxiety management approach.

The DARE Response is a lasting solution because it goes to the core of the problem, which is the resistance toward anxiety, and it heals by getting your anxious mind out of the way. It teaches you that you are not your anxiety. It teaches you that fear is just a feeling, thoughts are just thoughts, and you are truly safe.

So keep in mind that the core approach here is to never shun the anxiety or turn it away. When you slam the door on anxiety, it comes crashing through the window. So let it in and sit it down. Become comfortable with it.

I want you to even invite it to join you when you're not anxious at all! Send it a message to visit even on your good days. Keeping the door open for anxiety to visit stops you from worrying about it suddenly surprising you from out of the blue.

If you do this right, you'll feel a shift in your anxious sensations within just ten to fifteen minutes. The nervous discomfort starts to ease off and transforms into a kind of neutral, jittery energy, the kind of jittery feeling you get from drinking too much coffee. This is the kind of nervous energy you can work with and channel in a positive manner by using it to get things done. It's a positive and productive nervousness that makes you feel you can get up and go rather than paralyzing you with stagnant fear.

You may have heard that *fear* can actually be made into an acronym, FEAR, which stands for "Feeling Excited And Ready." That transformation is what The DARE Response enables if we accept our anxiety 100 percent.

ACCEPT AND ALLOW 100%

Acceptance followed by allowance is a very simple concept, but it can actually be quite hard to master. Most people get it wrong because they think they can just say the words *"Okay, fine, I accept you,"* and then their anxiety will magically disappear. They do it with the explicit intention of getting rid of the anxiety.

Unfortunately it doesn't work like that. Remember, The DARE Response is not about getting rid of the anxiety; it's about getting rid of your fear of the anxiety. At the risk of sounding trite, I'm going to repeat that point because so many people misunderstand it.

The DARE Response isn't about helping you feel calm and relaxed. It's not about making the unpleasant sensations go away. It's about ending your fear of the anxiety so that you can be free of it.

Be really okay with the fact that your mind and body might vibrate with nervous arousal all day long. Don't try to rush the wave of anxiety away. Let it move at its own pace. I know that new mindset isn't easy, but it gets you where you want to go.

Trying to force a state of calm is a type of resistance. It implies the following thought:

I really don't want this feeling, so I'll try to get rid of it with this exercise.

That's not how it works. I really want you to give up the idea of trying to be calm. What you're looking to achieve is to feel the sensations without getting upset or scared by them—to feel anxiety without getting anxious about it.

Allow the wave to pass and allow your nervous system to cool off in its own time without forcing the change. Let the anxious energy play itself out. Let it manifest in whatever way it needs to.

BECOME THE OBSERVER

This step of *allowing* your anxiety to be present is helping you to distance yourself from your anxious thoughts and feelings. You become a curious witness instead of a victim of your anxiety. You stop getting hooked in by each anxious thought or sensation and learn how to simply observe and allow it to be.

It takes training to get to this point, but soon you'll be able to experience all manner of uncomfortable anxious thoughts or feelings without feeling caught up in it. You occupy a new space of noticing and allowing. Things change from being *scary thoughts* to just thoughts, from *anxious sensations* to just sensations.

I don't mean to belittle how unpleasant the experience is, but remember it's all just a series of thoughts, feelings, and sensations. You're perfectly safe and no harm will come to you from it. Isn't it a relief to know that you no longer have to try to control anxiety? You can let it all flow through your compassionate acceptance and allowance of it.

But how will you know you're doing it right?

You'll know you're doing it right when anxiety manifests and you don't get upset or frustrated by it. You may still be somewhat scared of it, but you're no longer resisting the experience.

"Whatever!" you think to yourself as each anxious sensation jumps out at you. "*I accept and allow this anxious feeling. I accept and allow these anxious thoughts.*"

Welcome it all in and allow it to be.

STEP 3. *RUN TOWARD*

The previous two steps are the primary drivers that heal your anxiety. They propel you forward and often are enough to get you where you want to be. If, however, the anxiety still feels like a harmful threat hanging over you, you need to shatter that illusion by running toward it.

You run toward your anxiety by telling yourself you feel excited by your anxious thoughts or feelings.

Remember, anxiety is nothing more than a wave of energy flowing through your body. This energy will not hurt you. It's your interpretation of this energy that causes the problem and traps you in the vicious cycle of fearing fear.

Fear and excitement are just different sides of the same coin. When wildly excited, you experience the exact same sensations as you do when you're very anxious. The secret is learning how to flip your perception of these sensations from negative to positive. Once you master the ability to see them as nothing more than a heightened manifestation of energy in your body, you end the illusion of a threat.

Let the raw energy of your nervous system express itself fully. Let it excite you rather than terrify you. In clinical psychology, flipping one's perspective like this is called "arousal reappraisal." This is the conscious act of choosing to adopt a new perspective toward anxious bodily sensations.

A very famous clinical psychology study from the 1960s illustrates this point of perception perfectly.

Participants were told they were being injected with a new drug to test their eyesight. The participants were actually injected with adrenaline (which causes an increase in blood pressure and heart rate). One group were put in a room with an actor who pretended to get really excited by the drug; another group were put in a room with an actor who responded with frustration and anxiety.

As you might guess, the result was that each group responded in the same way as the actor in their group. So even though they all experienced the same nervous arousal, their perception of what was happening to them was directly influenced by the actor.

This study illustrated the point that it's not the bodily sensations we feel that trigger our emotional responses, but rather our *perception of those sensations* that determines our feelings.

If we reframe our perception of anxious sensations and move toward them skillfully, we become less intimidated or threatened by them. We achieve this very simply by saying

"I'm excited by this feeling."

Repeat that phrase several times until you feel a shift in how you're perceiving this nervous energy.

"I'm excited by this feeling."

Say it out loud if you're alone or to yourself if you're in the company of others. Stand up and bounce lightly from foot to foot just like an athlete does before beginning a race.

Choose to feel excited!

The idea here is to stop your brain from wrongly interpreting the sensations of anxiety as a threat and instead to trick your anxious mind into an excited state, the same kind of arousal you might feel if you were riding a roller coaster.

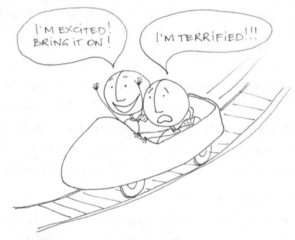

In essence, you're saying to your emotional brain: "This is not a threat. I'm not worried about this. It's just nervous arousal and I welcome it." Remember the acronym FEAR, "Feeling Excited And Ready."

In the beginning, you may have to fake it till you make it. That means that initially you'll find it hard to really run toward it and believe you're excited rather than scared, but with regular practice, the sensations that terrify you (e.g., a pounding heart, sweating palms, palpitations, dizziness, shortness of breath, queasy stomach) all become just that—sensations and nothing more.

Play around with this step and make it your own. Getting excited takes you off the fence and moves you directly into the sensations or thoughts that you fear. You are running toward the thing you fear most, and with this comes the realization that you are truly safe and that as uncomfortable as anxiety is, you can handle it.

STEP 4. *ENGAGE*

The fourth step in The DARE Response is short but crucial as it completes the whole movement from start to finish. It's designed to keep your anxious mind out of the way so that your nervous system can fully desensitize and relax back down.

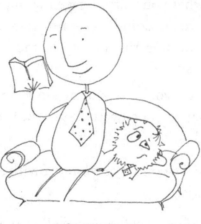

ENGAGE

After you've applied the previous three steps of The DARE Response, your anxious mind will naturally look for ways to reel you back into a state of worry and fear.

In order to avoid this, you need to engage with something that takes up your full attention. What that means is that once you've defused the initial fear and allowed the anxiety to be present, you should then ride out the declining wave of anxiety by occupying yourself with an activity that really engages your mind, anything at all that takes up your full attention, such as reading a magazine, focusing on a specific task at work, or having a conversation with someone in person or on the phone. Doing this keeps you in a state of flow and prevents you from getting hooked back into the anxiety loop again.

The most important point here is not to be idle. Idleness is the enemy of recovery. If you're idle, you'll ruminate and "check in" all the time. "Checking in" is that habit all anxious people have of scanning their mind and body to see how they're feeling every few moments. It's the anxious mind scanning for danger. You dramatically reduce the number of times you "check in" if you engage with something to occupy your mind.

Don't get upset when the anxiety keeps intruding. It will, I promise you—that's inevitable. So as it does, just keep gently placing your attention back on what you were engaged with and carry on in the full knowledge that you're doing everything right and that your new approach is in fact healing the anxiety in the background as you engage with other tasks.

For example, imagine you're sitting at work and suddenly feel a wave of anxiety. Maybe your heart skips a beat or your mind fills with anxious thoughts.

1. You immediately respond by *defusing* it with a playful "so what/whatever" attitude.

2. Then you move into *allowing* any residual anxiety you feel to be fully present. You get comfortable with your anxious discomfort. "*I accept and allow this anxious feeling.*"

3. Now *run toward* the anxious feelings by telling yourself that you are in fact excited by them. "I'm excited by this feeling."

4. Then finally, you move your focus back to what you were doing. In this case, you engage with the work in front of you without feeling a need to check in all the time because you know you're doing the right thing to heal your anxiety.

Please note there is a very subtle but key difference between engagement and distraction. Engaging with something is not a form of distraction. You're not trying to distract yourself from the anxiety; you're engaging with life again. You're allowing the anxiety to be present, but at the same time you're not going to stop living your life.

SUMMARY OF THE DARE RESPONSE FOR GENERAL ANXIETY

That concludes the four steps of The DARE Response. As a final comment, I would add that it's best not to overthink each step. Relax into it and try not to get worried about doing it perfectly (e.g., *"Am I doing it right? Should I try harder? Is it working?"*)

The most important thing is that you actually apply it each and every time you feel anxious. If after a few moments you feel another big wave of anxiety rise, then start The DARE Response over and go through the steps again. When you get very practiced at it, the whole process from start (step one) to finish (step four) will take only a moment or two. Eventually it will become second nature.

Think of The DARE Response as your special mental toolkit that you can use each and every time you feel anxious. By applying it (even imperfectly), you'll always be moving in the right direction and healing your anxiety.

To recap:

1. *As you become aware of anxiety, defuse it immediately with a "so what/whatever" attitude.*

2. *Drop all resistance and accept and allow the anxiety you're feeling to just be. Try to get as comfortable with the anxious discomfort as you can.*

3. *Remove the sense of threat by running toward the anxious feelings. Tell yourself, "I'm excited by this feeling."*

4. *Finally, move your attention to an activity in the present moment that engages you fully.*

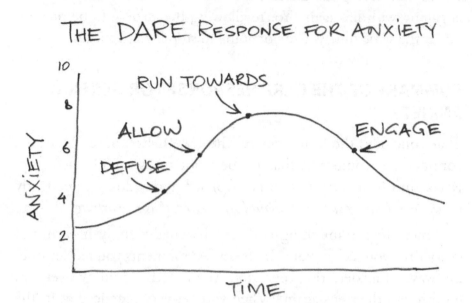

THE DARE RESPONSE FOR ANXIETY

The Science Behind The DARE Response:

 For those of you who are interested to learn about the psychology behind The DARE Response, please read the paper written by Dr. Joan Swart, PsyD in the appendix at the back of the book. Here is a brief summary:

Step	Right Move	The Tool	Objectives
1	*Defuse*	Mindful awareness	Awareness of automatic thoughts
2	*Allow*	Acceptance; Cognitive defusion	Allow unpleasant experiences to exist through cognitive defusion.
3	*Run Toward*	Cognitive reappraisal; *Paradoxical intention*	Reinterpret the meaning of the stimulus
4	*Engage*	Cognitive redirection	Reduce DMN activity and redirect attention and thought contents to focused goal-directed tasks

The DARE Response is applicable to all manifestations of anxiety. However, if *panic attacks* are your particular problem, you'll need to make a small addition to step three, which I'll explain in the next chapter.

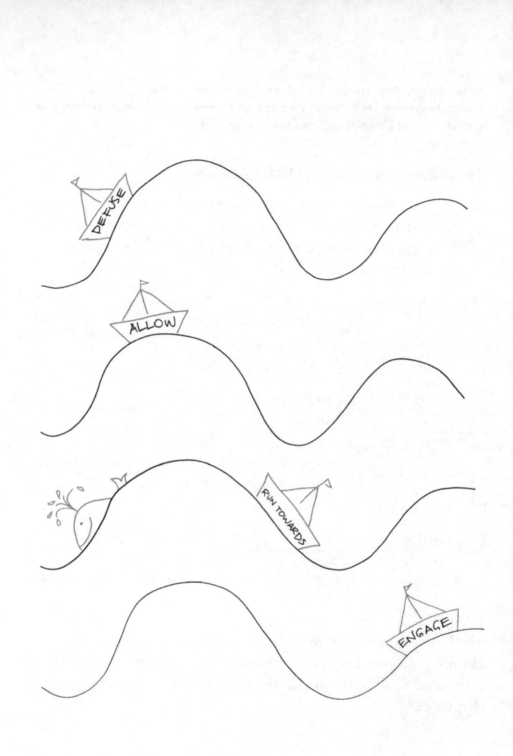

DARE

THE DARE RESPONSE
FOR PANIC ATTACKS

On a scale of 1 to 10 (where 10 is the highest), a person with general anxiety might score between a 5 and a 7, depending on the current life situation. When that person tops the scale around an 8 or a 9, they have what's known as a panic attack. These are very intense anxiety experiences. You'll absolutely know if you've ever had one. They're quite unforgettable!

Panic attacks are a false triggering of the fight-or-flight response. At the core of panic attacks is a type of catastrophic thinking that says, "This might just kill me." Panic attacks come on suddenly and usually include some of the following sensations or experiences:

- Pounding heart
- Sensations of shortness of breath or smothering
- Paresthesias (numbness or tingling sensations)
- Sweating
- Shaking

- Feeling of choking

- Chest pain

- Nausea / tummy cramps

- Feeling dizzy or unsteady

- An out-of-body or unreal feeling

- Shivers or hot flushes

Once we have our first panic attack, we immediately fear it happening again and begin avoiding situations that might trigger one. The fear of fear sets in, and the anxiety loop starts spinning.

Let me start by saying that if you suffer from panic attacks you need to understand that no matter how terrifying it feels, you are safe. No harm will come to you. You are not going to suffocate or die. Although it's very unpleasant, it's not dangerous.

There's an ancient Chinese phrase known as *zhilaohu* that translates as "paper tiger." It refers to something that seems threatening but is ineffectual and unable to withstand challenge. That is exactly what a panic attack is, a paper tiger—scary but actually harmless. (For a more detailed discussion on why these sensations are not dangerous during a panic attack, see the chapter "Give Up Fearing These Sensations.")

Dr. Harry Barry, an Irish medical doctor and expert in the area of mental health, has this to say about panic attacks:

"The job of your stress system is to keep you safe and alive not to kill you. The symptoms of anxiety are uncomfortable but they are not dangerous. You have my word as a doctor – this adrenaline rush will not kill you."

It's important to remember that panic attacks are not your enemy; they're the result of you trying to keep yourself safe. It's your ancient biological protection mechanism pumping you full of stress hormones so that you can fight a perceived threat or flee from it. This mechanism worked great when we needed to escape saber-toothed tigers thousands of years ago, but it's considerably less helpful when it's triggered while stuck in traffic or riding on the subway.

Think of all the panic attacks you've been through when the anxiety peaked and really scared you. Just when you thought you couldn't take it anymore, it settled back down again. Don't forget, your track record so far for getting through panic attacks has been 100 percent. That's pretty good.

Remember, anxiety arrives in waves. Every now and then, a really big wave will come (a.k.a. a panic attack), but if you don't respond correctly in those first few moments, the fear can swamp you, leaving you shaken and terrified of the next one.

The secret to ending panic attacks is to strip the fear away from the sensations that you feel. When faced with a panic attack, you need to run toward the anxiety with greater force. You do that by getting excited by the nervous arousal as explained in the previous chapter, and then you *demand anxiety to deliver more.*

YOU NEED TO *DEMAND MORE*!

You demand a more intense panic attack and really ride the wave of adrenaline out. Demanding more is the crucial addition to step three of the DARE Response because it allows you to run toward your fear and shatter the illusion of threat faster.

The request for more is the most empowering paradoxical move you can make when facing a panic attack. It's a request anxiety can't deliver. Your fear quickly subsides because the fuel that powers it (the fear of fear) has been suddenly cut off.

As Dr. Barry said, the rush or flood of adrenaline will not kill you. In fact, I want you to start thinking of panic attacks as nothing more than "adrenaline floods." The sensations that usually terrify you should be seen for what they really are: sensations of nervous arousal and nothing else. That's all you're experiencing: a pounding heart, sweating palms, dizziness, shortness of breath. That's it.

The actual fear you feel during a panic attack never comes from the sensations; it comes from *your response to those sensations*. The reason demanding more works is that it quickly short-circuits this false fear by proving once and for all that there's no real threat.

Demanding more sends a strong signal from the rational part of your brain (the prefrontal cortex) to the anxious part of your mind (otherwise known as the limbic system or the "emotional brain") that there really is no danger or attack. It's like a kill switch for fear. Your emotional brain gets the message and "click"—the panic alarm switches off and your nervous energy starts to discharge and unwind.

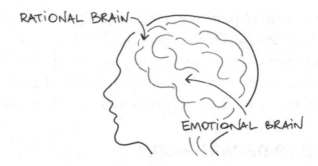

Your brain has now learned that *if* there really was a threat (e.g., if someone was in fact attacking you or you were being chased for your life), you would be too busy dealing with that threat—not demanding more of it!

Unfortunately today, most people are taught that the best way to handle a panic attack is to take some deep breaths and say reassuring things to themselves like:

"Don't worry. It's okay. Everything's fine."

But that kind of logical self-soothing doesn't work in the moment of panic; it's the wrong approach. Logic and reason get totally drowned out by the alarm your body is sounding. You have to get your emotional brain's attention by demanding more. That's the kind of crazy, counterintuitive move that gets attention.

Once you do this, your panic attack will discharge with a warm sensation as your anxiety level drops down to maybe a 7 out of 10. Now you can continue with the final step of The DARE Response: engaging with an activity in order to keep your anxious mind out of the way as the wave of anxiety subsides.

Here's an example of how this all ties together:

Let's say you're somewhere out of your safe zone and your heart suddenly starts pounding. "What's that?" you wonder to yourself. Then you begin to feel dizzy, or maybe your chest starts to feel a little tight.

You remember that the last time this happened you had a terrible panic attack and ended up calling an ambulance because you were sure you were going to die. That thought sends a shockwave of terror through your body, and more adrenaline is released.

Anxious "what if" thoughts now flood your mind:

"What if I have another really bad panic attack?"

"What if it never stops?"

"What if I collapse among all these strangers?"

With each "what if" thought, your anxiety escalates higher and higher until you have a full-blown panic attack. Before, you might have fled the situation to a safe zone or called someone for help. You would have resisted it. This time, however, you're armed with a new tool.

You begin to implement The DARE Response by responding:

"So what!" or "Whatever! This is just nervous arousal. I'll ride it out."

You close off the "what if" immediately with this quick response. Then you move into step two by accepting and allowing all the nervous arousal that you feel without resisting it or pushing it away. You welcome it in and begin to get as comfortable as you can with the anxious discomfort as you move along with the nervous arousal.

Now comes the new crucial step. If you feel the anxiety is not settling but rather peaking into a state of panic (8 or 9 out of 10), then you play your trump card, the one you've been holding in reserve for moments of panic. You chase it!

You tell yourself that you're **excited** by this feeling and **demand more** of the anxious sensations.

"I'm excited by this feeling! Give me more. Bring it on!"

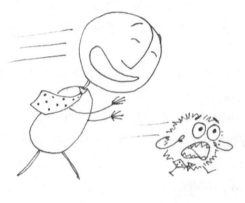

RUN TOWARDS

Talk to your anxiety and demand that it increase the intensity of the bodily sensations that scare you. For example, your heart's pounding fast, so you say:

"Okay, anxiety, that's good, but can you make my heart pound even faster?!"

You feel you can't catch your breath, so you say:

"Show me, anxiety, what it feels like if my throat and chest feel even tighter."

"I can feel a real knot in my stomach, but I wonder what it would be like if it were much tighter. Can't you make it tighter, anxiety? Is that the most you can offer?"

"I notice all kinds of fearful thoughts circling round my mind. Can

you make them more intense, anxiety? Aren't there any scarier ones? I've heard all these before."

THE ONLY WAY OUT IS THROUGH.

Bring it on. Demand to have a full-blown panic attack! *Become the hunter, not the hunted.* Let your anxiety know you're making a firm request, that you want to experience the very worst it can throw at you. Anxiety tries to convince you that you're in danger, but that's simply not true—so you call its bluff. This step is the paradoxical pinprick that pops the balloon of panic.

It's okay to be angry with the anxiety at this point. Say to it:

"You know what? I don't care anymore! Give me the strongest panic attack ever because I've totally had it with these false alarms ruining my life!"

"Bring it on <u>right now</u>. I'm no longer going to live in fear of this. OTHERWISE you better stop pestering me with this as I have a lot to do today."

"My life and the people in it are more important to me than any of these sensations, so do your worst because I've had enough."

Now you chase the anxiety, demanding that it show you more! That new mindset moves you from a state of panic into a state of power.

Do you remember in the movie *Forest Gump* how Lieutenant Dan battles the storm on the mast of his ship. "Is that all ya got?" he screams as the waves wash over him. The storm could not throw enough at him. When it eventually passed, he was a transformed man.

Demanding more may seem contradictory, but in life we often see examples of how acting in a very counterintuitive way is what is needed to get a desired result.

For example, when an airplane experiences a stall, it's frequently because there isn't enough wind across the wing to produce an adequate lift to hold the plane up. A rookie pilot might immediately pull the nose of the plane up in a panic to pull out of the fall, but that would only make matters worse. An experienced pilot, on the other hand, pushes the nose of the plane down hard into the fall instead of away from it. Anyone looking at him would think he was crazy to be pushing into the fall like that, but it's exactly what's needed to pick up speed and lift under the wings.

The solution here is the same. You need to make a forceful move into the wave of panic in order to ride it out correctly. You push in, to come out the other side.

Michelle Cavanaugh, who runs one of my coaching programs, likes to remind people of the kids' toy the "Chinese finger trap." Once you stick your fingers into it, good luck trying to get them out the traditional way! The harder you pull, the more stuck they become. To free yourself, you have to push into the trap in order for it to loosen—just like anxiety. You have to push in, to get out. You have to run toward it with force to be free.

I'm fully aware that some of you may be thinking:

"Whoa, no way! I'm not asking for more *panic sensations. If I call its bluff, it might just call my bluff back!"*

You fear that if you do in fact ask for more, the request will antagonize your system and create even more anxiety for you. But the wonderful truth is, *you have already had the worst panic attack you're going to have*. In the past your panic attacks have always peaked at a certain point then subsided. Once it passed, you may have spent days worrying about the next one or coming up with ingenious ways of avoiding situations where they might reoccur. But even in the worst panic attack, where you feared you were about to die, you never tumbled into an abyss.

You can trust this. You can trust yourself. You can trust in your own body's ability to handle the sensations. You can trust that you're safe. Getting excited and demanding more will not make matters worse. What it will do is change your relationship with anxiety back to its proper role as protector—not tormentor.

When done correctly, you'll feel the results instantaneously. That's why I sometimes refer to this step as a kill switch; you'll immediately feel a turning point as the adrenaline and cortisol stop flooding your system. You're then over the top of the wave. Some feel this turning point like a flushing heat sensation. If you feel that, it's a good sign. It's your blood returning to normal circulation.

As the anxiety leaves, which it will, wish it well and again keep the invitation open for its return. Yes, even invite it to come back!

You might say:

"Wait, come back. Have you nothing else to terrify me with?"

You need to welcome the anxiety to return in order to eliminate lingering thoughts of its unexpected return.

I know very well how unpleasant panic attacks are, and I'm not trying to pretend they're enjoyable experiences. *They are not.* But what I am trying to get you to see is that if you're going to experience a panic attack, then do it in a skillful manner so that the anxiety escalates no further. Allow the flood of adrenaline to run its course without your anxious mind stimulating more and more stress.

Up until now, panic attacks have been tossing you around, pummeling you with wave after wave of adrenaline. When you use The DARE Response, you ride up and over the big wave and then continue on with your day.

SHAKE IT OUT

Because there's a large amount of stress hormones in your system, don't expect to feel calm anytime soon. It will take a good twenty to thirty minutes for you to start to feel normal again as your body needs time to flush out all the stress hormones that were activated.

This is a good time to allow yourself to shake it out.

Many of us have the false idea that shaking means the anxiety is getting worse. Contrary to what most people think, shaking is actually a sign that your body is releasing the anxiety. It happens when the fight-or-flight response is winding down, not up! We need to understand that shaking is a positive thing. When we allow ourselves to express our nervous energy through shaking, we discharge it much faster.

Shaking is Mother Nature's way of de-stressing. In the wild, when an animal such as a gazelle has just avoided an attack, it will shake intensely for several minutes and then return to eating grass as if nothing happened. This shaking allows it to release the buildup of stress hormones that occurred during the attack. Animals don't need weeks of therapy; they just need to have a good shake to adjust back to life!

But we're not wild animals, and our culture frowns upon anxious shaking. Shaking is seen as a sign of weakness, so we suppress it. Instead, we tense up and hold ourselves in a rigid state. Not only should you allow your body to shake, but if you want to discharge your anxious feelings even faster, then encourage the shaking. Exaggerate it.

If you're sitting, tap your feet and bounce your knees more than you normally would. If you're alone, stand up and shake your body out. Shake your hands and arms. Shake each leg, then bounce on your toes like a sprinter before a race. Shaking helps to discharge nervous energy and rest your body faster.

SUMMARY OF THE DARE RESPONSE
FOR PANIC ATTACKS

1. If you feel the beginnings of a panic attack, respond to those initial waves of anxiety with a "**so what/whatever**." You're safe. Your body can handle it!

2. As the waves increase, *accept and allow* all the uncomfortable anxious thoughts and sensations to just be. Don't resist them. Bob up and down with them. Repeat to yourself, "*I accept and allow this anxious feeling.*"

3. If a wave of anxiety peaks into a panic attack, run toward it. Tell yourself that you **feel excited** and then call fear's bluff by **demanding more!** Ride up and over the wave of adrenaline.

4. Once the initial flood of adrenaline has passed, understand that there may be a few more minor waves of adrenaline to come—like aftershocks. Don't expect to feel calm anytime soon. You're going to feel on edge as the stress hormones slowly clear from your system. Allow your body to shake if it wants to and to complete the last steps of The DARE Response—*engaging fully* with an activity.

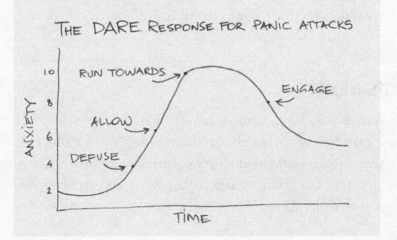

I know this can feel like a lot to remember, and some people say they can't think straight in the moment of panic. If that's your case, just try to remember this sentence, "Whatever! I'm excited by this feeling and I demand more of it!" Demand more of the thing that scares you, and the illusion of threat will quickly shatter. You'll reach a point where a panic attack starts, and your immediate response will be, "Let's do this!"

Practice and practice. If you don't get a result straightaway, keep at it. The more you practice demanding more, the more adept at it you'll become. Set little goals for yourself and get out there and push yourself to achieve them. Go to the supermarket if that scares you. Take that bus ride out of your comfort zone. Go for dinner with a friend. Set yourself small goals each day so that you can keep pushing into the panic and winning back your freedom. Put yourself in situations that trigger the anxiety to build your confidence faster. You then develop a deep faith that whatever comes your way, you can handle it. Your body can handle it. Your mind can handle it

Let this be your mantra:

"I can handle this."

Helpful Tip: Memorize this useful sentence in order to activate this step. "I'm excited by this feeling. Bring it on!"

"WHAT'S NEXT?"

The resistance you hold against anxiety can be very deep. There are also a number of myths about anxiety that need to be cast off because they create a drag that slows your recovery down. Over the coming chapters I'm going to teach you what you need to *give up and let go of* in order to move forward faster.

You'll find the philosophy of The DARE Response interwoven through these chapters. There will be some repetition of ideas, but that's necessary, as sometimes you have to consider a concept from many different angles before it really sinks in.

By the end of the book, you'll feel at much greater ease with your anxious discomfort. A sense of flow will return, and with that will come a renewed hope and optimism that you really can end your anxiety problem for good.

I wish that for you.

You're very close to feeling so much better.

Press on.

THE DARE RESPONSE

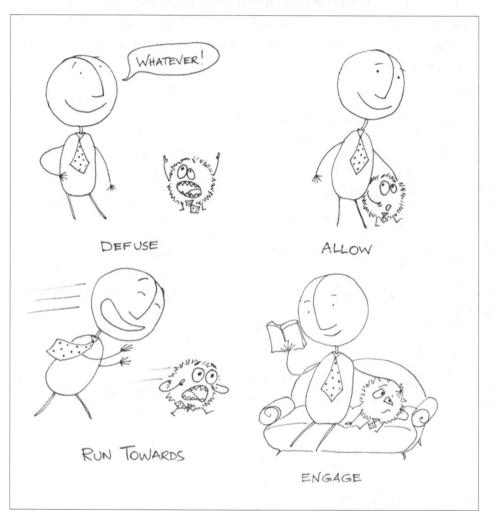

GIVE UP THINKING YOU'RE ABNORMAL

Anxiety is not a mental illness. Your brain is not broken. You are not going to go insane. I don't say this just to make you feel better; I say it because it's true.

The worst thing about anxiety is not how it feels physically, but rather the sneaky way it makes you think you're abnormal. Feeling abnormal is one of the most common experiences with anxiety. After experiencing high anxiety and stress hormones for a few months, almost everyone starts to fear for their sanity.

I bet at some stage you've felt like you're the only person in the world feeling the way you do.

"No one I know has these kinds of bizarre thoughts and feelings I have, so I must be mad, right?"

YOU ARE NOT YOUR ANXIETY

You'll have gathered by now that a key element of The DARE Response is to normalize anxiety as much as possible in order to escape its vicious cycle. Part of that normalization is learning to appreciate that *you are NOT your anxiety.* The anxious thoughts you experience are just thoughts and nothing more. They don't represent the real you. They're simply the result of stress hormones interacting with your vigilant and creative mind.

You are also not the only person going through this experience. Remember, according to the National Institute of Mental Health, some 40 million American adults alone (about one in six of the population), suffer from some kind of anxiety disorder at any given time.

Translate those numbers and you see that, as isolated you feel with your anxiety, you're not alone, and your experience is in fact very normal. When you're out and about, reflect on that "one in six" statistic. You might have been thinking that no one else could be dealing with your particular anguish, but look again. That woman serving you breakfast might be fending off a panic attack. The irritated man in front of you in the bank might hate the claustrophobic sense of waiting in line. The mother driving the SUV might be afraid that she'll have a panic attack on the highway with a car full of kids.

Anxiety is such a common problem, yet not one talks openly about it. The subject of mental health is still a taboo subject. Our celebrities happily talk on national TV about their colon cleansing or their sex lives, but rarely do they mention their mental health. That seems to be too personal, the topic too vulnerable.

With over 50 million yearly prescriptions written for just one antianxiety drug, alprazolam (the generic name for Xanax), isn't it time we started to talk more openly about anxiety in particular and how common and normal an experience it is? If we could normalize the whole experience for society through the mass media, I think far fewer people would fall into the anxious trap of fearing fear.

A DOUBLE LIFE

Has anxiety caused you to lead a double life?

I hazard a guess that to the outside world you pretend that all is well while inside you fear you might lose your mind. A bit like a secret agent, you guard this secret from the world. I bet very few people would even suspect you have a problem with anxiety at all.

Isn't it amazing how we can continuously portray one image to the world while inside we feel completely tormented? Women are good at this, but men are the grand masters of hiding anxiety away. I know all about that because I too used to be one of those secret agents.

Someone once remarked to me, while I was going through a particularly rough phase with my own anxiety, that I seemed as laid back as a duck floating down a stream. What they never realized was that underneath the water this duck was paddling like crazy just to stay upright.

A few years ago I was coaching a very well-known TV presenter who was plagued by the fear of having a panic attack live on TV. He was terrified that his colleagues might suspect something, so every day he entered the studio he plastered on a smile and acted as if nothing could faze him. He kept all his fears and anxieties to himself for years. He didn't even tell his own wife about the daily torment he was going through every time he went on air.

I bet you're an incredible actor. You pretend to the world that all is well and then secretly spend the day dodging and weaving any situation that might make you anxious. That double life is exhausting. You might have one or two close friends who suspect something because you frequently avoid certain situations, but by and large the rest of the people in your world don't suspect a thing.

Flying is a good example of how well people hide their fears. Statistics show about 30 percent of all passengers on any given flight are nervous about flying and about 10 percent are extremely anxious—but it's hard to spot those 10 percent during a flight. They sit tight and secretly grip on to their armrests until their knuckles turn white—all without making a peep. They're going through sheer terror but hide it well because of an even greater fear, the fear of shame. The fear of humiliation.

Anxiety and shame can play off each other in an almost comical manner. For example, let's say you're having lunch with some work colleagues. Suddenly your heart skips a beat and your chest tightens. In a split second you convince yourself you're about to have a heart attack BUT instead of asking them to call for an ambulance, you excuse yourself politely and make for the bathroom. *You would rather die alone from cardiac arrest in a toilet cubicle than cause a scene.*

I think you'll find that whenever you place the fear of humiliation above your fear of imminent death, anxiety is surely at play!

TOXIC SHAME

Anxiety is a deep-seated source of shame for most people, and shame is a toxic feeling that keeps us stuck in the experience of an adrenaline flood and delays our full recovery. In order to begin healing our anxiety, we have to give up our sense of shame about it. If we expose it to the light of day, we'll see it for the lie it is.

Shame manifests in different ways for anxious people: Shame of being weak. Shame of failing as a mother or a father or a boss or a friend. Shame of not being able to support your family and provide an income. Shame of not being able to be out of your safe zone or go shopping alone without your safe person.

Most of this shame is driven by negative self-talk. For example, a father dealing with anxiety might think: *"How can I, the man of the family, not be able to take my kids to a ball game?"*

A college student might think: *"Everyone else is so outgoing, yet I'm afraid to sit for even a few minutes in a lecture hall."*

A new mother might think: *"I have this amazing child that I cherish so much, but these anxious thoughts are stealing all the joy I should be feeling. How can I think such things? Am I a terrible mother?"*

There are some people who don't hide their anxiety and seem happy to talk about it, but even then the conversation tends to be at the surface level. If you dig a little bit deeper, however, you'll inevitably find that same shame lurking in them, shame they don't want to share with anyone, things they don't want to admit to for fear of being judged.

Often the shame cuts very deep indeed. I got a call once from a woman who wanted to talk about her panic attacks and constant anxiety. She lived with her husband and kids in a small town. She told me how anxiety and panic attacks were destroying her quality of life, and every day was turning into a pitched battle. She used to travel all around the world for work as a sales executive for a large corporation, but she now found it hard to step out the front door for fear of having a panic attack.

I asked her if she had told anyone else about her anxiety problem besides her husband and doctor. She responded that she had let a few friends know, but in general she kept it to herself, fearing others might start to gossip about it. I then asked her what it was that really troubled her the most about her anxiety.

She got a little irritated and said, *"Haven't you been listening to me? I can't leave my home because of this, and I have kids to look after. What could be worse than that?"*

"No, I get that," I said. "But what REALLY troubles you about your anxiety?"

There was a long silence. Then after a moment she said, "Not leaving home is just the half of it. The other stuff I could never admit to anyone. ... I'm too ashamed."

"Well, try me," I said. "I'm pretty much a stranger, just someone at the other end of a phone line. I don't imagine we'll ever meet in person. You have nothing to lose."

"Okay …," she said. "So deep down I fear I'm losing my mind. Like I'm losing touch with reality. I'm never present with my children because the whole time I'm thinking about my anxious thoughts."

I told her that people can often admit to their doctor or close friends about their panic attacks or general anxiety, but they rarely admit to the things that really upset them the most. They hide their greatest fears so deep and suffer in terrible silence.

It's normal, for example, for such people to be afraid to pick up a kitchen knife in case they go nuts and stab someone or to get anxious behind the wheel of a car for fear of swerving uncontrollably into coming traffic. Or they hate to stand out on a balcony in case they suffer a moment of madness and jump off. Other shameful, anxious thoughts revolve around forbidden, aggressive, or perverse sexual thoughts or doubts about one's own sexual identity.

So many people suffer silently from these types of intrusive, anxious thoughts, and I wish they all had a chance to understand how very common they are. Such thoughts are very common and are not a sign of mental illness, but rather a result of high anxiety, stress hormones, exhaustion, and an overactive imagination. That's it. (I discuss these types of intrusive thoughts in the chapter "Give Up Fearing Anxious Thoughts.")

I'll share an incident one man told me which really summarizes the kind of shame people with anxiety disorders suffer from. Tom, who suffered from frequent panic attacks was the father of a ten year old boy. Every weekend he would berate himself for not having the courage to do certain things with his son. Things like going fishing or camping, like he used to do when he was growing up with his father.

On one occasion shortly before we spoke he described a recent outing to a pop concert. They were going to see a popular band play in a local venue with a few of his son's friends and their parents. Tickets were not cheap and his son had been looking forward to "this cool gig for the longest time." They were sitting several rows of seats in when Tom started to feel the uncomfortable tight chest sensations that usually triggered panic attacks for him. He tried to ignore it as best as he could but as soon as the band came on stage and the crowd began to roar he felt his anxiety spike and needed to get out of there. The problem was, they were all there together and the sense of being trapped with these people in the venue only made his anxiety worse. He lasted another few minutes but then suddenly stood up and told his son to follow him outside. As they left he explained to the other parents that his son was not feeling well and that they were going to go home. This surprised the others as his son had been in a great mood all evening.

When they got outside his son's eyes welled up with tears as he asked his father, what was wrong? Why had he lied? Why did they have to go home?

Tom didn't know how to respond and just mumbled something about an urgent thing he needed to do, as they walked quickly to the car and then drove home. The whole incident filled Tom with such a deep sense of shame that it affected his core sense of self-worth.

LETTING GO OF THE SHAME

In order to end any shame, you have to unmask it. You have to admit it first clearly to yourself. You need to be clear in your own mind about what it is that you could never admit to another. Then the healing can start. Shame is a lie that doesn't serve you in any way. When you expose it to the light of day, it loses its grip on you because it's exposed for what it is: an illusion.

There is no shame in suffering with an anxiety problem. You're in good company. Some of the greatest minds in the world are believed to have suffered from anxiety, including the scientists Charles

Darwin and Sir Isaac Newton. Famous artists and writers such as Alfred Lord Tennyson, T.S. Eliot, Marcel Proust, Emily Dickinson (the list is endless), are all believed to have suffered similarly.

The link between creativity and anxiety is well established. Research shows that people who suffer from an anxiety problem tend to score higher than average on intelligence, creativity, and sensitivity. What happens, unfortunately, is that all those positive characteristics can turn in on themselves when stress and anxiety manifest. A sharp, intelligent mind rushes to diagnose all unusual physical sensations, and when it draws a blank, the anxiety takes over and jumps to irrational conclusions. Deepak Chopra wrote, "The best use of imagination is creativity. The worst use of imagination is anxiety." The sensitive personality with a creative streak often uses its imagination to come up with scary scenarios straight out of a horror movie. How often have you felt a sensation and then let your imagination run riot with everything imaginable that might be wrong?

THE MECHANICS OF ANXIETY

To further help you understand and normalize anxiety, let's take a closer look at what actually causes anxiety and the bodily sensations associated with it.

I'm sure most of you have heard of the fight-or-flight response, coined by Walter Cannon. This is at the core of your stress response. As I mentioned earlier, this is an automated survival mechanism that has enabled mankind to survive in a very harsh and dangerous natural world. If a saber-toothed tiger crossed your path 8,000 years ago looking for its lunch, your body's survival mechanism would have flooded you with adrenaline so fast, you could have escaped in a flash (if you were lucky).

The interesting thing about the fight-or-flight response is how it takes over complete control in that moment of danger. The conscious brain is not consulted; everything is about immediacy. You hear stories where people jump out of the way of oncoming traffic or perform amazing physical feats—such as lifting up an automobile to rescue someone trapped underneath—when this response is suddenly activated.

Operating the fight-or-flight response is the limbic system, a complex set of brain structures that lies in the middle of your brain—what is also referred to as the "emotional brain." The amygdala is a central part of the limbic system, and it sets the whole series of events in motion by sending a red-alert message to the hypothalamus to fire up the nervous system and prepare for danger. The adrenal glands above the kidneys are then instructed to release adrenalin and cortisol into your bloodstream.

You know very well exactly what this feels like. It's an unmistakable feeling when adrenaline is flooding your system. BOOM! All of a sudden you feel pumped and either highly excited or highly anxious. Note that adrenaline by itself doesn't make you feel scared; it just makes you feel really aroused and alert.

Remember: what causes the problem is your interpretation of the stress response. When you learn to change your interpretation (response) using The DARE Response, you change the way you experience stress and anxiety.

The fight-or-flight response happens in a split second. The impact of these hormones is felt immediately as your heartbeat and breathing increase. Your blood is drawn away from routine functions like food digestion and pumped into your muscles so that you can get out of there fast or stand and fight your threat. As all of this is happening, your muscles contract in preparation for an attack, and your bowels and bladder relax. It's all an incredibly and ingenious biological response to keeping you safe from harm.

The fight-or-flight response is a survival mechanism designed to keep you safe from a threat, and "threat" is the key word here. In your case, the problem is almost always never a real threat. You just sit down to get your hair cut and BOOM! Off it goes. Or you get in your car and as soon as you encounter traffic on the freeway, BOOM! Another flood of adrenaline is triggered by your emotional brain.

There's no real threat, but your body is acting like there is one because you're sending the message that there is danger.

Take the example of having to give a presentation or a public speech. Your logical brain knows a speech won't kill you. No one is going to physically threaten you on the podium, but your emotional brain is responding to the fear of being judged and socially ostracized.

Your emotional brain has not evolved to decipher between real danger and imagined threats. You can actually trick your brain quite easily into believing an imaginary thing is real. For example, imagine for a moment you're sucking on a piece of lemon. Think of that for just a moment and your mouth begins to produce saliva. The lemon is imagined, but your brain has led your body to think this experience is real and to respond appropriately. The same applies to fear. Your emotional brain imagines a threat then hijacks your rational brain and takes over the show. Your body's response follows in a very real and physical way with the fight-or-flight response.

Let's look at some of the typical bodily sensations of the fight-or-flight response. Understanding these in detail will help you normalize each and every one of them so that you can implement The DARE Response easier.

1.   Pounding heart

If you were truly threatened, you wouldn't even notice your heart pounding in your chest. You'd be far too busy fleeing to safety, and even if you did notice it, you'd expect it to be pounding. When you watch a scary movie or are about to do an interview, you know that a pounding heart is normal. But what if you can't identify any reason at all for your pounding heart? Then your mind rushes to the conclusion that a pounding heart must mean something is wrong.

This is probably the single-greatest cause of concern for people. As soon as the fight-or-flight response is activated and no threat is identified, most people then rush to the conclusion that they're having a heart attack. Why wouldn't they, right? Their hearts are beating like crazy for no reason, and they're having all the bodily sensations we associate with a heart attack (e.g., pins and needles, chest pain, dizziness). This is why so many people end up in the hospital ER claiming they're having a heart attack only to be told later it was just anxiety. (Please note: you should of course always get your heart checked if you have any concern about it, even for peace of mind.)

2.   **Increased breathing**

When you're anxious, your rate of breathing increases. Immediately your anxious mind rushes to the conclusion that something is wrong, and you try to take control over your breathing. What a job to take on! The more you try to manage your breathing, the more uncomfortable you feel. This quickly increases your fear and anxiety as your mind plays all kinds of scenarios, such as having to go to the hospital and have a machine manage it for you. The other negative side effect of all this is that there's usually a slight drop in the amount of oxygen and blood sent to the brain, which can lead to feeling dizzy and confused. In extreme cases of overbreathing, you can feel extreme pins and needles in your arms and hands, even to the point of hand cramps where your thumb and fingers close together (carpopedal spasm). This is not dangerous, but it is, of course, very distressing.

3.   Excess Nervous Energy

If you were to run from or stay and fight a real threat, all the excess nervous energy created by adrenaline would dissipate easily. With an unidentified threat, however, you don't move, and that nervous energy lingers in your system longer than it normally would. This can make you feel uncomfortable for an extended period of time and also make you shake or feel very jittery and on edge. You want to get up and walk around, get outside, or be on your own. Sometimes that's possible, but if you're in a situation where it's not easy to excuse yourself, you start to feel claustrophobic, and you get more anxious, creating more adrenaline.

4.   Muscles tension/tremors

As you prepare for fight or flight, your muscles tense, particularly in the neck and upper body. With no physical exertion, this tension lingers in your muscles for way too long, leaving you feeling uptight and stiff. You may also notice that your muscles shake or that you have tremors in reaction to the adrenaline in your system. You may feel your legs start to shake or even witness your entire body shaking like a leaf.

5.   Sweating

Sweating increases during fight or flight in order to keep you cool when running or fighting a threat. The main negative side effect of this during a false alarm is the social embarrassment that comes with it. If your fight-or-flight response is triggered by a social event like having to give a speech or do an interview, excessive sweating can make you feel even more self-conscious and anxious.

6.   Dizziness

The dizziness felt during an episode of panic or anxiety is often caused by increased respiration. You tend to overbreathe (hyperventilate) when you're anxious, which can lead to dizziness or lightheadedness. Passing out when highly anxious is very rare because fainting is the result of low blood pressure. When you feel anxious, your blood pressure goes up, not down. Hence, fainting is unlikely because your brain has plenty of blood supply.

7. Bowels and bladder loosen

When experiencing anxiety, you'll likely feel the need to go to the bathroom. This is one of the more bizarre features of the survival response, but it's thought to occur in order to make running away easier as you'll carry less weight! The big side effect of this today is the abject terror of soiling yourself in public. This is extremely uncommon, but you may have this phobia that manifests as a fear of not being near a bathroom. This is a fear that's more common in women.

8. Digestion and salivation slow down

The reason you feel butterflies in your stomach when the fight-or-flight response is activated is that the digestive system is shut down and blood is drawn from your stomach area and sent to your muscles and other vital organs. The problem with this is that it can lead to feelings of nausea, a very heavy feeling in your stomach, and a fear of vomiting. Again, if you're out in public, this can easily feed into a social anxiety. The other area that slows down is saliva production, leading to the uncomfortable sensation of dry mouth.

9. Anticipation/ Worry / Derealization

The fight-or-flight mechanism puts your brain on alert to anticipate all possible threats as well as those that have not manifested yet. This is why it turns inwards when it fails to find an external threat. Like a hound dog, it's on the trail of all possible threats and tries to seek out where the next threat might come from. If you're continuously anxious, this turns into chronic worry or the "what ifs." Eventually a "worry about things" becomes a "worry about thoughts" where you worry about the very contents of your mind and fear you're going nuts.

There is a very particular sensation not often mentioned in other literature called derealization that occurs after a person has been suffering from general anxiety for some time. It's a sense of unreality, as if all the world is an illusion. This sensation causes people to feel very abnormal and is one of the more unsettling sensations associated with anxiety. I discuss it in more detail in a later chapter, but suffice to say it's not harmful, and once the general anxiety level is reduced, this sensation ends.

DON'T BUY INTO THE LABELS

As mentioned previously, I try to avoid using the word "disorder" when talking about anxiety problems because I think it encourages people to buy into a label when an assortment of symptoms could be evidence of a wide variety of situations and resolved in very different ways. If the goal is to normalize anxiety, we need to demystify it and not get lost in the clinical jargon mental health professionals are so fond of.

Remember that anxiety is a temporary problem. Do not define your life by it. You are not a label.

> *"But my problem is very complex! My doctor told me I have 'OCD with generalized anxiety disorder and a sprinkling of panic disorder to boot.'"*

Yes, you may well have all the symptoms and behaviors that fit neatly into the clinical definition of an anxiety disorder according to the DSM *(American Psychiatric Association's Diagnostic and Statistical*

Manual). But when you zoom back out, you'll see the core problem is one and the same, anxiety manifesting in various ways. It all falls under the same umbrella, and healing it is brought about with the application of the correct approach.

I can appreciate why the medical community uses these labels. It's the nature of science to reduce symptoms and behaviors to distinctive categories so that they can better understand them. The trouble is that such cold diagnostic labeling has an impact on how people perceive themselves. Vulnerable people can leave a doctor's care thinking that this label assigned to them is now who they are. What's worse is that there is a huge amount of subjectivity when people are diagnosed using the DSM. Although rates of consistency have improved, the diagnosis of mental health issues, like anxiety disorders, remains very much more of an art than a science.

My heart goes out to all those people who seek a solution to what they're experiencing and all they get is a diagnostic label and a long-term prescription for medication. These people leave the doctor's office feeling even more abnormal than when they walked in the door!

The goal of this book is to do the opposite for you. It's designed to teach you that even though you're having these very uncomfortable and strange experiences, you are in fact totally normal. When you learn to normalize your experience of anxiety, you heal it much faster.

In closing, let me reiterate the point I made at the start of the chapter. You are not your anxiety. As abnormal as it makes you feel, this anxiety is not the real you. It is not who you are or who you have become. Once your anxiety level starts to drop through the application of The DARE Response and the stress hormones are slowly flushed from your system, you'll start to feel a whole lot more like your old confident self again. Trust me on that.

GIVE UP SAYING NO TO ANXIETY

"The bamboo which bends is stronger than the oak which resists."

-Japanese proverb

One of the hardest steps of The DARE Response for most people is the second step: the idea of dropping resistance and really allowing and accepting the anxiety. The goal of this chapter is to help you achieve that by teaching you to move more fully with each anxious wave of anxiety.

My family used to have this great dog called Shadow. He was a cross between a collie and black Labrador. He used to sit all day long in the front room of our house waiting for anyone to come to the front door. When someone would finally arrive, he'd go absolutely bonkers!

Until … we invited the person in.

If we kept the person at the door (for example, the FedEx guy), Shadow would bounce off the walls, barking loudly with all the hair on his back standing straight up. No matter how hard we tried to tell him to lie down and stop barking, he wouldn't listen.

His reasoning was: *"I'm the guard of this house, and if my owner doesn't invite a person in, then that person is unwanted and therefore a threat."*

I sometimes used to keep friends standing at the door for a few minutes and then let them in (if they were brave enough), just to see the change in Shadow's reaction. It was the same every time. Once they passed the front door, he'd immediately stop barking and sit back down on his seat.

Anxiety is just like a guard dog. It's your protector. It's your fight-or-flight response activated by the emotional part of your brain, designed to keep you from harm. It needs you, the owner (your rational brain), to reassure it that the unusual bodily sensations that pay you a visit are not a real threat and that all is well.

But as we've seen, just saying, *"Everything is okay. Calm down now,"* doesn't work. Just like Shadow, anxiety responds much better to your actions. You need to mentally allow the anxiety in. If you keep the door on anxiety closed, your emotional brain thinks that the threat is real and there is something to be afraid of. When you invite your anxious sensations in with total acceptance of them, your emotional brain (your guard dog) backs off and calms down.

Charlotte Joko Beck says, "We have to face the pain we have been running from, in fact we need to learn to rest in it and let its searing power transform us."

I love the way Beck expresses what's at the very core of real acceptance: *to rest in it and let its searing power transform us.*

Learning to rest in anxiety is the way you heal it. Resting in the uncomfortable sensations gives your mind and body a chance to relax and detoxify from the stress response. So when you feel fear or anxiety surface, instead of pushing it aside, whisper to yourself, "It's okay." Give a gentle "yes" to the moment and what you're feeling. Acceptance of the anxiety brings a sense of peace and understanding that all will be okay in time.

Nobody wants to feel anxious. Who would? It's a really uncomfortable, unsettling experience. But not wanting to experience anxiety isn't going to make it any better or make it go away. Frustration and stress are all that comes from wishing things were different than they are. The way you feel right now is the way that it is. *You don't have to love your anxiety. You just have to permit it.*

Dr. Carl Rogers wrote, "Acceptance is a pre-condition of change." Acceptance of your current state is your freedom from it as it allows for a positive change to happen. Saying "yes" to anxiety opens you up to the energy and vitality that are behind the anxiety so that you can transform it from something fearful into something positive.

"I accept and allow this anxious feeling."

When you say "yes" in this way, you increase your tolerance of anxious sensations. With this heightened tolerance, the tension you feel is reduced and eventually eliminated. As a side effect, you end up getting what you want. You end up feeling calm. The anxiety leaves *not because you forced it away* but because you're no longer fueling it with resistance and fear. Saying "yes" is the very essence of The DARE Response.

Please don't think that saying "yes" to anxiety is about giving in or surrendering to it. Saying "yes" is a statement of empowerment—not subjugation. This is about you calling a truce to the civil war you've been waging against yourself. Saying "yes" comes from the powerful and grounded you.

I know that it's easy to agree in principle with saying "yes" to anxiety, but it's much harder to implement. When you use this approach, you have to pay attention to your thought processes as you engage with your anxiety. Many people think they're saying "yes" when in fact they're still saying "no." They're willing to take a few tentative steps toward the anxiety, but they're scared of it swamping them and therefore hold back and never really do it 100 percent.

Let me give you the example of Christine, whom I was speaking with recently. Her anxious sensations are a lump in her throat and dizzy sensations. She fears she might faint when she's outside her home, even though she's never fainted before.

She said to me, "I'm trying your approach to stop the anxiety, but it's not really working. It's not going away. What am I doing wrong?"

I drew her attention to her choice of words: *"trying your approach to stop the anxiety ... It's not going away."*

I explained to her that to really do The DARE Response correctly, she has to stop saying "no" to the anxiety and ease herself into the anxious discomfort. She can't hide from it or try to stop it from happening. In Christine's case, that means she needs to go to the places where these sensations manifest (at the shopping mall in her case) and sit there with them—not push them away, but become the observer of them and get comfortable in the anxious discomfort.

I explained to Christine that pushing these sensations away or trying to "make them stop" is not acceptance of them. She needs to allow them to be present and say "yes" to the anxiety all day long.

"Come on, lump in the throat! Let's go shopping. Hey dizzy spells, you're coming with us too!"

When you *attend and befriend* you move yourself out of fight or flight. That's what saying "yes" is really about. That stops the inner friction and allows your thoughts and emotions to flow with the waves of anxiety that you feel. It isn't about pretending to like the sensations. It's about having an open and embracing attitude toward them. This attitude allows you to now go places and still have a good time regardless of whether the sensations are present or not.

Christine found it hard to accept the sensations initially because she feared allowing them in would only cause them to get worse. Maybe you feel the same way? Maybe you fear that inviting in and befriending the thing that scares you will only cause you to go over the edge. This is where you'll have to really trust me and this process.

You've already experienced your worst anxiety episodes. What's been happening since then is that you're keeping that anxiety locked in place with your resistance to it. This resistance is the quicksand that's keeping you stuck. When you stop saying "no" and drop the resistance, you gradually pull yourself out of the muck.

I think the process of accepting anxiety is a bit like learning not to scratch an itch that really irritates you. In the beginning, the itch is all you can think about and you keep going back to scratch it to get some relief. Scratching the itch of course just makes it worse, and you then become obsessed by the irritation it's causing you. Through acceptance, you eventually learn to sit with the discomfort of the itch without scratching it. You focus on your day and allow the itch to be there without scratching it. It's not easy to do, especially in the early stages, but slowly the itch starts to be less of an irritant, and you notice it less and less until eventually it's gone.

The same thing happens when you accept and stop resisting your anxiety. You're no longer responding to it in a negative way. Your brain eventually filters it out, and you no longer notice its presence. As soon as you stop responding to it in fear, you stop fueling it and set yourself free from its discomfort.

It's not that you'll never have anxious sensations again. They'll manifest from time to time, especially when you're stressed or exhausted, but you now have a default way of responding to it. You say "yes" to it. I've already made reference to the fact that battling anxiety is like having a tug-of-war with your anxiety. The more you pull against it, the harder anxiety pulls back. The tension and friction you feel comes from the rope that you're holding so tightly. You fear letting it go in case you lose the battle. *By learning to say "yes" to the anxiety, you drop the rope and the resistance.*

IT'S OKAY TO FEEL SCARED

Anxiety can be a really scary experience. Allow yourself to feel scared if that's how you're feeling. Allow yourself to feel vulnerable. The more you allow yourself to just accept the way you are right in this moment, the faster the charged emotion of fear will dissipate. Remember, the wave rises and falls. *These are just thoughts and feelings. They can't hurt you.* The only power they have over you is the power and meaning you give them. So give them no significance or meaning. Normalize them and let them pass.

Embrace the anxiety without any judgment and without opinion. Say "yes" with a smile and allow yourself to feel whatever manifests. If you do this 100 percent, the feeling will shift within a few moments into something else. Sensations change from moment to moment. It won't be gone, but it will transform into a more tolerable feeling simply by saying "yes" to it and allowing it space.

Allowing all uncomfortable thoughts and emotions their space is key. There's a popular metaphor of the blue sky obstructed by grey clouds. It comes from mindfulness teachings, where you imagine your mind is like the bright blue sky and your anxious feelings are like dark clouds that roll in. No matter how many dark clouds appear, the bright blue sky is always there in the background watching. The blue sky allows the dark weather to come and go no matter how unpleasant it looks. Eventually the bad weather passes, and you're left with the bright blue sky again.

Acceptance and allowance of what is takes practice. In the beginning, you'll certainly feel the urge to say *"No, I don't want this."* You'll feel the storm brewing and think, *"I don't like the look of this,"* or *"I don't want to feel this."* That's a natural response, so just allow that thought of resistance to come up, observe it, and *allow it to be present as well.* All storms pass. The dark grey clouds of anxiety will drift away faster if you allow them space to do so.

You might also have some resistance coming up toward this book and me. You will question if I really know what I'm talking about. You'll have thoughts about dropping this approach and going back online to find some other solution that asks less of you. Allow that resistance to simply exist as well. Give it space and just observe it. Smile inwardly as you know this is just a game between you and your anxiety.

Saying "yes" puts you back in your flow, which is an open, soft, and compassionate attitude toward all the things that you feel. It's like a cool stream of water that calms your nervous system. It shifts you from a state of "fight or flight" to one of "rest and digest".

In her excellent book *Hope and Help for Your Nerves,* Dr. Claire Weekes wrote about flow by using the concept of *floating* with anxiety. The DARE Response relates to that same concept that she wrote about over fifty years ago. You float (or flow) with the nervous arousal, and in so doing, the anxiety is diminished.

When you flow with your anxiety, the dark clouds quickly pass and are replaced by blue sky. If you do this right, you'll be surprised by how fast the anxious feelings and sensations change. But remember, don't look for that change or try to force it to happen. Allow it to happen in its own time. The paradox of healing anxiety is that you're attempting to generate a positive change while simultaneously being okay if that change doesn't happen right away. Crazy, right? But that's just the way it is.

Here's how a client of my coaching program put it:

"What has been bothering me about my progress, and about the whole program is that it does seem paradoxical: 'OK I will accept you so I can be rid of you!' I am really good at realizing that I am actually safe, and that the sensation won't hurt me. What I haven't been that good at is going along with the sensations. Now I see that I just have to go along, doing whatever I need or planned to do, while having the sensations and not so much distract myself from them, but just not give them space in my head."

ALWAYS BE PLAYFUL WITH THIS APPROACH

Say "yes" to the anxiety with a playful attitude. That can mean having a humorous running commentary with yourself and a smile on your face as anxious thoughts and feelings rise up from out of nowhere.

Another client described that running commentary like this:

"I get great results when I joke with my anxiety: 'Ahhh there you are, or there is that bodily sensation that usually scares me ... how interesting. I wonder what scary thoughts are going to now come along with that sensation? Come on, Daffy Duck and all your scary thoughts, don't hide. I am not going to bite. I just want to see you. I am not going to get frustrated with you or run away from you. In fact do you want to spend some time with me? I am going into town now so why don't you come along for the ride.'"

Each time the anxiety pulls at you, attend and befriend it. Smile inwardly and say, *"Yes, you're welcome to come in. Take a seat. I'll be with you in a minute."*

If anxiety continues to pull at you with frightening "what if" thoughts, think, *"Okay. Whatever. I hear you. You can stay, but I have this thing I have to finish, so I'm just going to do that. I'm not pushing you away. I just don't think this is as urgent as you (anxiety) are making it out to be."*

Toward the end of my own recovery, I used to get these random waves of anxious thoughts that felt like a punch to the stomach. As soon as I felt these, I knew it was time to say "yes" and implement The DARE Response. I would start by reminding myself not to resist any of the thoughts no matter how alarming they were, but rather embrace them all.

Before, the old me used to scream, "NO! Not now!" Then, sure as day, a huge wave of anxiety would suddenly pound me, and I would think, "NO MORE!!!!" and whoosh, another 40-foot wave would hit me. Wave after wave of fear and anxiety would slam-dunk me to the point where I was lost in a sea of adrenaline and fear. Once I learned The DARE Response and how to say "yes" instead of "no," these waves of fear and anxiety soon became nothing more than small ripples.

FLASH FEAR AND RESPONSE FEAR

There are two types of fear connected to anxiety. Dr Weekes calls them first and second fear. I call them "flash fear" and "response fear." Flash fear is a wave of intense sensations. This fear is so immediate and sudden that you have no control over it. Response fear is your response to the initial flash fear. The DARE Response is about training yourself to now have the right response to flash fear.

Response fear is where all the trouble starts. It's where the anxiety loop begins and where your suffering comes from. If you didn't have any response fear, all you'd have would be brief moments of unusual sensations that would flash momentarily on your consciousness. I believe everyone has flash fears all the time, but they don't develop into a problem (a disorder) because they aren't followed by any great amount of response fear.

When your general anxiety level is stuck at a high level, you'll frequently experience these flash fears: those moments when you have a sudden, scary thought followed by a jolt in your nervous system. It can also manifest as a strange feeling that flashes over you while you're chatting to someone or busy at work. Maybe it's a sudden sense of impending doom, apprehension, or unreality. They can also be triggered by a memory of a past situation. These flash fears happen with such immediacy that you have no control over them.

Flash fears can also be very physical (e.g., your heart suddenly starts pounding, you feel dizzy, or your stomach knots). Your fight-or-flight response has suddenly been activated for whatever reason. These are sensations that happen so fast you have no immediate control over them.

Next comes your response. Up until now, it's been one of fear, an immediate wave of flash fear that comes without warning. Response fear, which comes next, however, is something you do have control over. It's something you actively do even though it also happens quite fast.

Response fear is the "what if" thinking that says:

"What the f*** was that? Oh no … is something terrible going to happen now?"

"This happened before and I ended up in ER. I'm about to have another panic attack!"

Response fear feeds off the flash fear through "what ifs" and quickly escalates into a state of high anxiety. What started off as an uncomfortable bodily sensation has turned into a full-blown panic episode through response fear. If flash fear is like nibbling the bait, response fear is falling for the lure—hook, line, and sinker. This is why the very first step in The DARE Response is to defuse these "what if" flash fears as soon as they manifest.

Everyone experiences flash fears to some extent. The difference is that a person with high anxiety experiences them with greater frequency and more intensity than a person who's not particularly stressed. Complete acceptance of all flash fears is crucial. I am fully aware that training yourself to have the right response to flash fear is difficult. In the beginning your initial response will still be the wrong one; that is just habit. As long as you immediately correct it though, you prevent it from spiraling out of control, and you will get the desired result. Eventually the correct response will become automatic and second nature to you.

I bet in the past, you used to experience the same flashes of anxious bodily sensations that scare you now. Back then, though, you didn't pay them too much attention as you weren't in a sensitized state. They simply didn't register on your radar. Now, however, you're highly sensitized and attuned to every sensation. You have your "anxiety radar" set to maximum alert and pick up on absolutely everything: every little hiccup, every heartbeat out of place.

By applying The DARE Response and saying "yes" to anxiety, you start responding to anxious sensations much like you did before this was ever a problem. You don't respond with fear. You slowly begin to relearn that there's nothing wrong with you to begin with!

GIVE UP FEARING THESE SENSATIONS

Anxiety and panic are fueled by a fear of sensations. In order to really move out of an anxious state, you need to stop obsessing and fearing the anxious thoughts and sensations that scare you. In this chapter on sensations, I include *physical* sensations, such as a pounding heart or a tight chest, as well as *mental* sensations, such as intrusive thoughts or derealization.

I want to help you give up your fear of sensations by shedding light on the most common sensations associated with anxiety and demonstrate how you might apply The DARE Response to them. Throughout, I want to emphasize the importance of relaxing your response to these sensations and then learning to get comfortable in the anxious discomfort they create.

Remember: ***recovery is never about the absence of sensations***. Full recovery is when you reach a stage where sensations manifest, yet you pay them no heed. You can go about your day-to-day life and not be concerned whether they're present or not. That's when anxiety is no longer a problem for you. Thus, you see anxiety is *not in the sensations; it's in your resistance to the sensations.*

Let me give you an example. We don't get anxious about a pounding heart just after we've been running because we know the exercise was the cause of the sensation. Nor do we get anxious after having stubbed a toe. The problem comes when we can't identify a cause for the sensation. Our brains are designed to keep a vigilant lookout for threats in order to keep us safe. If we feel a strange sensation and don't know why it's manifesting, we tend to jump to fearful conclusions.

Just to give you an example of that, scratch your head with your fingers right now. Listen closely to the sound it creates. Now, imagine you don't know what's causing that sound. Wouldn't you start worrying that something horribly wrong was happening to your head? The higher your general anxiety level, the more you overreact to unknown sensations.

Another example I like to give of how our minds rush to fill in the gaps is of a man who told me he once took his wife's car to work and got into a panic when he suddenly noticed a very strange sensation in his feet. He was feeling quite anxious at the time, and this unusual sensation triggered the start of a panic attack. He then glanced down to see that the air conditioning of the car was set with the cold airflow directed toward his feet. The air was causing the unusual sensation. He burst out laughing and realized for the first time how oversensitive he was to unusual bodily sensations. It helps to emphasize the point that anxiety isn't in the sensations; it's in our resistance or response to those sensations.

"Recovery lies in the midst of all the sensations you dread the most."

-- Dr. Claire Weekes

I'm going to teach you how to apply The DARE Response so that you may have a non-anxious response to any bodily sensations, regardless of whether you know the cause of those sensations or not.

As you read about each sensation in this chapter, you may very well find yourself experiencing them to some degree. If that's the case, don't worry—on the contrary, welcome them. It's only when these sensations are present that you have an opportunity to practice having the right attitude toward them.

I have listed below some of the typical sensations associated with anxiety and panic. These are common offenders, but there are many more not listed here that you may experience. If you have sensations that aren't listed here, you'll nonetheless get a very good idea of how to apply The DARE Response to them by reading through the examples given.

In this and the following chapter ("Give Up Fearing These Situations"), you don't have to read through each example given. You can skip ahead to the ones most applicable to you. After each sensation, I'll go through each of them and discuss how The DARE Response applies in that particular case. It goes without saying that any sensation causing you concern should be investigated by your doctor to rule out possible causes other than anxiety. Doing so is not only important from a medical point of view, but it will also help reduce anxious thoughts that something more serious might be wrong.

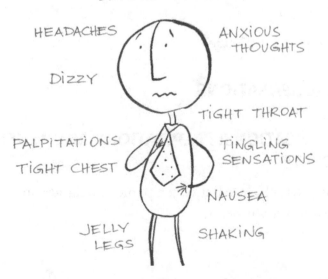

DEPERSONALIZATION

HEADACHES

DIZZY

ANXIOUS THOUGHTS

TIGHT THROAT

PALPITATIONS
TIGHT CHEST

TINGLING SENSATIONS

NAUSEA

JELLY LEGS

SHAKING

PHYSICAL SENSATIONS

- *Heart Sensations: Palpitations and Missed Heartbeats*
- *Breathing Anxiety*
- *Fainting/Passing Out*
- *Nausea/Fear of Vomiting*
- *Choking Sensations/Tight Throat*
- *Headaches*
- *Blurred Vision*
- *Weak Legs/Jelly Legs*
- *Shaking/Tremors*
- *Tingling Sensations*

MENTAL SENSATIONS

- *Losing Control*
- *Unreality/ Depersonalization*
- *Disturbing Thoughts*
- *Depression*
- *Fear of "Going Crazy"*

PHYSICAL SENSATIONS

HEART SENSATIONS: PALPITATIONS AND MISSED HEARTBEATS

Most people who have experienced panic attacks at some point fear for the health of their heart.

If you're worried about heart problems you should certainly get your heart health checked out if for nothing else than to put your mind to rest and reduce the effect of anxious "what if" thoughts.

When you do get a clean bill of health, trust in the results and don't second-guess them. If you really must, get a second opinion, but after that—stop doubting your good health.

The major symptoms of heart disease are breathlessness and chest pain as well as occasional palpitations and fainting. Such symptoms are generally related to the amount of physical effort exerted, i.e., the harder you exercise, the worse the symptoms get.

Let's take a quick look at some common heart sensations before examining how you might apply The DARE Response.

PALPITATIONS

Palpitations are short, abrupt periods in which the heart suddenly starts beating fast. If you're in a sensitive state, this can ring alarm bells because you fear a sudden heart attack. The more you panic, the faster the heart beats. It's therefore understandable why you might jump to conclusions in this situation and call for medical help. What you have to remember is that palpitations are perfectly natural and can often be caused by exhaustion or stimulants like caffeine. Your heart is an incredibly strong muscle, and it won't stop or explode simply because it's beating hard and fast. A healthy heart can beat fast all day long and not be in any danger.

MISSED HEARTBEATS

The medical term for missed heartbeats is extrasystoles. A missed heartbeat is usually the result of an extra beat between two normal beats. Because of the pause that follows this extra beat, it can seem as if one beat was missed. And because the heart's lower chambers fill with a greater-than-usual amount of blood during the pause, the next regular heartbeat can feel like a bit of a jolt. When you feel this sensation, you often freeze and wait in terror to see if your heart's in trouble.

Such missed beats are generally harmless. It can help to sit down when you feel this sensation, but if you wish to keep moving, do so. Exercise won't cause the situation to get worse, and don't convince yourself that going home to lie down is the only way to help the situation. If you retreat every time you feel an unusual sensation, that behavior can reinforce a negative idea that your home is the only safe place to be. Your heart is not an atomic clock that must always keep perfect time. It speeds up; it slows down. Occasionally it beats in an irregular fashion. From time to time, you may notice an irregular beat or two. This is nothing to get upset about.

The New England Journal of Medicine recently published a study by Dr. Harold Kennedy who found that healthy people with frequent irregular heartbeats appear to be no more prone to heart problems than the average population. The majority of even the healthiest people experience palpitations, missed beats, or pounding in the chest.

You can convince yourself that if you worry enough about your heart, or concentrate too much upon its actions, it may somehow get confused and forget how to beat correctly. It's quite common for people who suffer from this type of anxiety to check their pulse at regular intervals to make sure it's beating correctly. You need to be aware that no matter how much worrying you do about it, your conscious mind can't stop your heart from beating. All it can do is speed it up for a period of time through fear and anxiety or slow it down marginally through mental relaxation exercises.

How to apply The DARE Response

When you experience a heart sensation, be it a pounding heart, palpitations, or missed heartbeats, first **defuse** the "what if" fear immediately. Tell yourself:

"So what if my heart doesn't stop beating so fast?"

"Whatever. I know my heart's in good health and can more than handle this."

The important thing is to **defuse** the initial "what if" fear and then **allow** your heart to beat in whatever rhythm it sees fit. Place your awareness there and don't try to control the natural rhythms of your body by always insisting on a calm and steady heartbeat. The more you allow your body to flow in the manner it so chooses, the faster it will return to a state of rest. The more comfortable you are with the diversity and range of your heartbeats, the less likely you'll be to overreact with anxiety when it happens. Trust that your body has this incredible innate intelligence and simply telling your heart, out of fear, that it might stop beating doesn't mean that it's going to pay attention!

If your anxiety about your heartbeats is escalating into a sense of panic, **run toward** that fear by getting excited and demanding more of the sensation. For example, if your heart is pounding, try mentally to get it to pound harder. If you notice a skipped beat, try to bring on another one. After a few moments of this, your fear of the sensation will lessen, and you can go back to allowing the sensation to be without wishing or forcing it away.

Once you've defused the fear and allowed the sensation to be present, the next thing to do is to **engage** with something that grabs your attention. Try your best not to keep focusing back on your heart or checking your pulse.

Very often, your heart only wants to palpitate a bit, thump a few beats harder. Why? That's the heart's own business. It's your anxious mind that gets upset and panics, causing the adrenaline to kick off a longer cycle of rapid heartbeats. So from now on, make a verbal agreement with your heart that you're going to stop interfering and obsessing over its health. You're going to trust it 100 percent. Just allow your heart to be, place your awareness there, and let it behave in whatever way it wishes to behave. By allowing the sensations to happen and then engaging your mind with an activity, you release the anxiety that you hold around your heart and reduce the constant monitoring of every heartbeat.

As you get more comfortable with the sensation, you'll find just answering the initial "what if" thought with the response "whatever" may be enough to stop any further anxiety from manifesting.

BREATHING ANXIETY

It's common for people with anxiety to mention fears about their breathing. Some feel that their breathing is very labored and shallow. These fears are almost always accompanied by a sensation that feels almost like a tight band around the chest. Some people worry that they're not getting enough oxygen or that they might stop breathing altogether, and this causes them to feel forced to take conscious control of their breathing. One client described this sensation by saying it felt like living on a planet that didn't have enough oxygen.

The chest or throat tightness that causes uncomfortable or shallow breathing is very common. It's often triggered by esophagitis (inflammation of the esophagus caused by acid reflux). When the esophagus is burned by refluxed acid, these nerve endings fool the brain into feeling short of breath, as though the lungs were not providing enough oxygen. Other causes can be due to muscle tension in the chest area, giving the sensation of reduced respiratory capacity. As always, you should get a full examination to determine the cause of the problem. You can then treat the physical issue (e.g., esophagitis) while at the same time using The DARE Response to reduce your anxiety about not getting enough air.

A tight chest or fears about not getting enough air progress quickly to "what if" thoughts about suffocating or fainting from lack of oxygen. Don't let this worry you. Believe me, you could spend every minute of the next ten years worrying that you'll stop breathing—and nothing would happen. What a waste of your time and energy.

Your body knows exactly what it needs, and even if you try with all your mental might to get in the way of it, your body will still breathe. Your respiratory control center has a reflex mechanism that will eventually force you to breathe if you're not getting enough oxygen. You simply can't override it with your anxious mind. All your fear can do is change your rate of breath.

Many people experience this sensation every day, but they don't panic because they don't have a high level of sensitization and general anxiety. You may notice yourself that on some days you have these sensations but they don't trigger anxiety or panic—and they quickly pass away, proving once again that anxiety is *not in the sensations, but in your resistance to the sensations.*

How to apply The DARE Response

When you become overly conscious of your breathing and the "what if I stop breathing/suffocate" thought fires off, **defuse** this fear by answering the question with a powerful "so what/whatever."

"What if I suffocate?"

"So what? At least I'll have a good excuse for not showing up at my in-laws' dinner party tonight."

Of course, you don't really mean it; the point is to be humorous and flippant with the threat in order to make light of it. Come up with responses that suit your own sense of humor.

Remember, you won't stop breathing just because you're worried about it. Tell yourself that it's fine for the muscle tension and shortness of breath to be there. **Allow** it to be there. You're not worried; it can stay as long as it likes. It's not a problem because there's no threat to your safety.

Say to that part of your body:

"That's fine. I accept and allow this uncomfortable sensation around my chest. It can stay, and I'm going to continue with my day."

If you feel that your breathing is too shallow, allow it to be shallow. If you feel you can't catch your breath, then just allow that sensation too. Your body always compensates as it adjusts to expel excess carbon dioxide. The point to remember here is that your breathing is an unconscious process, and your body has always—and will always—look after that for you, regardless of how much your anxious mind gets upset about it. The more you can sit with the sensation and not respond with fearful thoughts, the better. The more comfortable you get with the sensation, the faster the sensation releases.

If you find that you simply can't stop worrying about your breathing, **run toward** the fear more forcefully by telling yourself you feel excited and demanding your chest feel even tighter or your breathing get even shallower. You can really push into the fear by exhaling all the air in your lungs and holding your breath just to really prove to yourself that your breathing will look after itself. Then, once it starts to settle, go back to allowing the sensation without mentally wishing or forcing it away.

When you feel ready, **engage** with something that really demands your full attention in order to keep your anxious mind out of the way and to stop obsessing over your breathing.

This fear is a perfect example of how your anxious mind can get in the way of a natural flow. When you learn to trust again in that natural flow of your body, you stop interfering and worrying, and a comfortable, natural rhythm returns to your body. Reestablishing this trust in your body's natural rhythm and ability to handle stress is fundamental in recovery from anxiety.

FAINTING/PASSING OUT

When you experience high anxiety or panic, it's very common to feel lightheaded or dizzy. This sensation is alarming because it makes you feel very vulnerable. If you're alone, you might fear falling unconscious with no one to look after you. Or if the sensation happens in public, it can lead to feelings of vulnerability while surrounded by strangers.

The dizziness often felt during an episode of anxiety is caused by increased respiration. People tend to overbreathe (hyperventilate) when they're anxious, which can lead to dizziness or lightheadedness. Dizziness can also be triggered by pressure to perform in situations.

For example, you may think:

"I don't know why, but any time my boss asks me a question, I freeze up and start to feel dizzy."

Certain situations can also trigger anxious memories, like this:

"I felt dizzy the last time I was in an elevator; now every time I get in one, I start to feel a bit woozy."

It's extremely uncommon to faint when feeling anxious or threatened because fainting is the result of low blood pressure. When we faint, the body falls to the ground. This allows blood to be supplied easily to the brain, a clever safety mechanism. When you feel anxious, your blood pressure goes up, not down. Hence, fainting is unlikely because your brain has plenty of blood supply.

Think of situations where people are faced with imminent threats, such as a robbery or major catastrophe. People don't faint left, right, and center. They always respond with a heightened sense of alertness because their bodies have been primed to jump into action by the adrenaline released into their systems. Their hearts beat faster, their breathing increases, and their blood flows fast. This prehistoric response to threats has been with us since early mankind. If cavemen fainted every time they saw a predator, mankind would have had a very short history!

Quite simply, fainting when anxious is highly uncommon due to the amount of blood that's being circulated. Your heart is usually beating fast, so there's little worry that the brain would be short of a fresh supply. Frequently what happens is that people who have fainted in the past tend to be particularly frightened by a dizzy spell because they feel that if it happened before, it's likely to happen again.

If you've fainted before and fear it might happen again, try to remember the circumstance you were in: Were you tired? Was the temperature very hot? Had you eaten correctly that day? Fainting can be the result of many different factors. Generally, it has little to do with anxiety and is more frequently associated with energy levels, diet, and temperature.

If you struggle with this fear on an ongoing basis, you need to disempower the fear. Here's how.

How to apply The DARE Response

The next time you feel lightheaded or dizzy and the "what if" thoughts of fainting flash in your mind, **defuse** them with a resounding "so what" or "whatever!"

"If I faint, I faint and there's nothing I can do about it. Within a minute I'll come back around."

If you feel very dizzy, it's important to find a place to sit to help you get your bearings, and always pull over safely if you're driving a car.

You then **allow** your body complete permission to be dizzy. If your head wants to spin, let it. If you see stars, that's okay.

If the fear of fainting continues and it feels like it's pushing you into a state of panic, **run toward** this sensation. **Demand to faint!**

Tell your anxiety:

"If you're going to make me faint, then let's have it now. But if not, then sorry, but I have to keep going and get on with my day."

No one can faint on demand. You won't faint just because you demand it. What you'll find is that the fear evaporates quickly as you call its bluff.

You can then gently begin to **engage** with something that will hold your interest for longer and longer periods of time. As the anxiety lessens, continue your focus on an activity that will keep you from worrying constantly about the dizzy sensation coming back. If the "what ifs" keep popping up in your mind, repeat the above steps.

With all sensations (dizziness included), try not to leave the situation you're in, or you may start avoiding that situation. Stay where you are and work through it until the anxiety subsides.

NAUSEA/FEAR OF VOMITING

Anxiety has a direct impact on the abdominal region. It can make people feel anything from a mild jittery sensation (butterflies in the stomach) to physically sick. Most people tend to get more anxious when they imagine they might vomit, which worsens the sensation of anxiety, thus making it all the more likely to happen. The fear of getting sick makes the situation worse. This fear is driven by "what if" thoughts like:

"What if I get sick right here and now? What would I do? What would people think of me?"

It's more common for people to fear vomiting in social settings than when they're at home because they think they don't have a safe place to retreat to and will instead feel exposed to social embarrassment.

How to apply The DARE Response
Defuse these "what if" thoughts fast.

"So what if I vomit? I have a paper bag here and I can use it if I need to. No big deal."

Then **allow** the sensation in your stomach to manifest in whatever way it wants to and give it full permission to be present. Tell your anxious stomach that it's fine to feel sick, and if it feels it's necessary to vomit, then it may do so and you won't try to stop it. The reason this approach works well is that as soon as you allow your stomach the freedom to feel uncomfortable, your abdominal muscles immediately start to relax and you feel less nauseous.

If you feel you are still worried about vomiting, **run toward** the fear and tell yourself that this feeling in your stomach is just a result of nervous arousal, like butterflies in your stomach, and that you are excited by this feeling.

Overfocusing on a nauseous feeling only keeps you feeling tense, so it's best to then **engage** as best you can with anything that will keep your attention off the sensation in your stomach.

In the early stages, while you're learning to apply this approach, I do recommend you carry a small paper bag with you (like the ones found on airplanes). The bag reassures you that no matter what happens you can deal with it.

You likely now get the idea of how to apply The DARE Response for any sensation that makes you anxious. To avoid repetition going forward, I won't outline The DARE Response for the sensations below, but instead I'll just add some additional tips on how to handle the sensation.

CHOKING SENSATIONS/TIGHT THROAT

Anxiety can cause a tight sensation in the throat that people often describe as a lump in their throat. The medical term for this is globus hystericus. This sensation is the result of muscle tension in the throat area. Although uncomfortable—and at times upsetting (the *hystericus* in the name is related to the word *hysterical*)—this sensation is not harmful.

For people who experience this in association with eating, I find that it's the thought of forcing a swallow that causes them to feel anxious.

If you feel very uncomfortable while eating, the best approach is to simply chew your food and make no attempt to swallow. Just keep chewing. You'll find that you can't stop the process of swallowing— it's a natural reflex. By not feeling that you have to force a swallow, the pressure is off. Swallowing happens as a natural reflex if you simply keep chewing. You can have fun experimenting with this. Try to eat anything at all and force yourself not to swallow. It's almost impossible. This is a great approach for people who fear swallowing because they don't have to put themselves under any pressure to swallow. When pressure is removed from the equation, the problem solves itself.

I believe a lot of people experience a lump in the throat due to a buildup of emotion. During emotional events, such as weddings and funerals, it's common to feel this sensation. And what's more interesting is that, when people express themselves (e.g., crying, laughing, talking), the swell of emotion dies down and the sensation ends.

So if you feel this sensation on a regular basis, I suggest that you start singing or humming. Singing or humming to yourself for several minutes on a regular basis releases the muscle tension in the throat area. For this to be most effective, focus on the singing, not on trying to see if the sensation has gone. Like many other anxiety sensations, the less you preoccupy yourself with it, the faster the issue is resolved.

Some might associate this "lump in the throat" sensation with a disease. In practice, real lumps in the throat, such as a cancer, are not always felt. (This is one of the reasons that a tumor can get so big before it's discovered.) Nevertheless, if you're concerned about your throat—or any other part of your body—always get a full medical examination. This is the fastest way to put anxious "what if" thoughts to rest.

HEADACHES

If you experience high anxiety or stress, it's very likely that you also experience headaches, or even migraines. Some describe their headaches as dull pain or a tight band around their heads. A migraine is a headache that is experienced in more severity, sometimes associated with sensitivity to light, sound, and movement. If you work in an office, the artificial light—such as from computer monitors and televisions screens—might trigger a migraine. In fact, migraines in association with anxiety are very typical in office settings.

The most common of all the various headache types is a tension headache. This is caused by a tightening of the muscles in the upper back, neck, and head. Researchers in Taiwan have found that the majority of people, particularly women, with chronic daily headaches have either anxiety or depressive disorders. Anxiety can make tension headaches worse by increasing muscle tension from the stress response.

There are many possible cures for headaches, including short- and long-term solutions. Your doctor is best able to advise you on how to treat your particular headache or migraine.

BLURRED VISION

When frightened or anxious, the pupils in the eye dilate quickly, and this can sometimes cause blurred vision. Blurred vision can also occur when looking quickly between near and far objects because the pupils change dimension.

Blurred vision is also often caused by fatigue or when the eye muscles start to lose elasticity with age. Even though anxiety can frequently cause instances of blurred vision, it's important to visit your doctor for an eye checkup. For example, if the blurred vision occurs with a discharge, it may be conjunctivitis and need treatment. If something needs treatment, early detection can often result in correcting the problem.

WEAK LEGS/JELLY LEGS

Anxiety creates the sensation of weak or "jelly" legs. When anxious, adrenaline is released into your body. The adrenaline can make sensitive people feel very weak in their muscles—especially the leg muscles because they're supporting the body. You often hear people say that when they have to stand up and speak, they go weak at the knees and fear they might topple over. It's important to note, however, that the jittery sensation you may feel in your legs is not a signal that your legs are any weaker—they're not. On the contrary, your legs are being primed for movement, so don't fear that they'll go out from under you.

If you're out walking and you feel this sensation, continue to walk; if you're standing in a line, continue to stand. There's no need to find a place to sit, and doing so often reinforces your anxiety about weak legs. If you train yourself to continue to do what you were doing, you'll quickly learn that the sensation of weak legs is an illusion and your legs are strong and very capable of supporting your body. The more you challenge anxious sensations in this manner, the faster the sensation will disappear. Many anxiety symptoms are worsened by anxious thoughts about the sensation. For example, if you feel your legs go weak, you may jump to extreme conclusions, such as:

"Weak legs mean I'll fall over—and that means I must be about to faint!"

When you think like this, the anxiety can then trick you into feeling dizzy, thereby creating an even greater cycle of anxiety. The answer, as you're now well aware, lies in first accepting the sensation with a "so what/whatever" and then allowing it to be. Allow your legs to shake as it helps discharge the nervous energy you feel faster.

SHAKING/TREMORS

It's really common for your body to shake or for you to feel minor tremors in your legs and arms when anxious. As previously explained, this is particularly common after a panic attack. Shaking is to be encouraged, not suppressed. Allowing yourself to shake allows you to release the buildup of tension in your muscles faster. To speed this process up, you can shake your arms out and jump from foot to foot.

TINGLING SENSATIONS

When panic attacks begin, people often feel a tingling sensation in their body. The medical term for this is *paresthesia*. More generally known as the feeling of pins and needles, it's a sensation of tingling, pricking, or numbness of the skin, and it has no apparent long-term physical effect. Paresthesia is most commonly felt in the hands, arms, mouth, and feet. Don't be alarmed—this is perfectly natural to experience in connection with high anxiety. Once your anxiety level drops down, this sensation will pass.

MENTAL SENSATIONS

It's important to understand that anxiety causes a type of mental exhaustion. In this section you'll learn that mental sensations, such as obsessive or intrusive thoughts or fear of losing control, are just signs of this mental strain or exhaustion and not signs of a neurotic illness. You can apply The DARE Response for mental sensations in exactly the same way you do with physical ones.

For example, with each troubling mental sensation you'll want to:

Defuse the anxious "what if" thought as soon as it appears.

"What if I go insane and they lock me away?"

"Ah well, whatever. At least I won't have to cook dinner anymore, and I can catch up on some reading."

Then **allow** the anxious thought to manifest any time it wishes. Invite it to stay as you go about your day without reacting in fear of or resistance to it.

If the sensation is causing you a sense of threat, **run toward** it. Get excited and demand more of that sensation.

Finally, **engage** your mind with something so that you don't start obsessing over the thought too much or giving it too much of your attention. At the end of this chapter, I've included more thoughts about how to use The DARE Response for mental sensations.

SENSATION OF LOSING CONTROL

During a panic attack or experience of high anxiety, some people are prone to believing they're going to lose control. This feared loss of control can be physical (e.g., that all your vital organs will completely lose the run of themselves and descend into chaos) or emotional/mental (e.g., that you'll lose your grip on reality, and it will never return). Those who hate social embarrassment tend to suffer from this fear the most. The feared loss of control could range from screaming in public to smashing their car into a guardrail on the highway.

Put your mind at rest! As scary as those thoughts may be, you're not going to commit any of these acts. The reason you experience these thoughts is that your body feels out of control due to the constant bombardment of stress hormones in your system. Your mind thinks that if your body is out of control, it's next on the list.

You're not going to lose it. In fact, I'm sure that with all the panic attacks and heightened anxiety you've experienced in public places, nobody even noticed that you looked uncomfortable. We are, by nature, social animals, and we dread being seen in some kind of embarrassing situation. The idea of jumping from your chair and screaming for an ambulance during a business meeting may go through your mind, but it's unlikely to happen. Most people find a way to politely excuse themselves. In the end, even if you do embarrass yourself socially, does it really matter? You have to learn to be kind to yourself. So what if you cause a scene and great embarrassment? Life's too short to keep up with appearances all the time. In fact, the more honest you are with your fears, the less pressure you subject yourself to.

UNREALITY/ DEPERSONALIZATION

The sensation of unreality is often cited as the most disturbing and uncomfortable sensation associated with anxiety. Psychologists call this sensation derealization or depersonalization disorder (DP). Suddenly there's a change, and objects and familiar situations seem strange, foreign.

Many people who experience panic attacks and constant anxiety become distressed by this sensation and feel they may be losing their mind. They report feeling disconnected, as if separated from the outside world by a fog or pane of glass. This often leads to believing that some permanent damage has been done to their brain, which is causing these sensations.

A typical manifestation of this depersonalization or unreality is when you're having a conversation with someone and you suddenly feel alarmingly isolated and removed from the situation. Once this sensation arises, it can be so impactful that it sticks with you for days, and worries about its return keep popping up. It's difficult to accept that such a disturbing symptom is simply a result of high anxiety, but it is.

The sensation is caused by two things: delayed perception and mental preoccupation. While under constant stress or anxiety, the buildup of stress chemicals in your system causes a delayed response in sending information between neurotransmitter sites in your body. This slight delay between experience and thought can create a momentary sensation of unreality.

The same effects are experienced under the influence of marijuana, but people don't react with fear because they're aware that the drug is causing the sensation. When DP occurs as a result of a bad drug trip, it doesn't cause long-term damage, but individuals must avoid whatever drug triggered it as further episodes are likely if they take that drug again. It's when the sensation arrives while you're just talking to someone at the water cooler at work that things feel a little scary!

To this day, little is known about depersonalization, but one theory states that depersonalization is a protection mechanism your brain uses to keep you from experiencing trauma. This sensation is often associated with high-intensity traumatic events. In order to protect you from the emotional impact of that event, your brain in effect numbs you by using a *psychological anesthetic* if you will. People who experience panic attacks or high anxiety could be triggering depersonalization as a protection mechanism in response to the trauma of the intense anxiety they experience.

I mention depersonalization because the condition isn't often discussed, and I want to reassure those of you who may have experienced it that it absolutely will pass as soon as your general anxiety level reduces—trust me on that. Once the mind and body return to a normal level of relaxation, your body then has the opportunity to dispel some excess chemicals, and the sensation of being disconnected from the world ends. It's very easy to start imagining all the terrible mental illnesses that this sensation could mean, but don't worry. You haven't caused any damage to yourself, and you'll soon return to the person you were before depersonalization crept in.

The quickest way out of this disconnected feeling is to apply The DARE Response and then allow time to pass. Don't fight or resist it. **Defuse** the "what if" thoughts that you have about the sensation being a sign of some serious mental problem. It's not; it's simply the result of high anxiety.

Then get comfortable with this very uncomfortable sensation by **allowing** it to be. If the sensation is causing you a sense of threat,

run toward it and discharge that heightened fear of DP by telling yourself you are in fact excited by the feeling it creates. Tell it you want even more of the same! Of course, this is not true, but it allows the fear to discharge faster. Finally, **engage** your full attention with an activity that keeps your anxious mind from obsessing over the uncomfortable DP sensation. The **engage** phase of The DARE Response is crucial with DP as it's the constant obsessing over how weird everything feels that keeps it present.

Engaging with activities such as strenuous walking, running, biking, swimming, etc. are some of the best options as physical activity gets you out of your head and into what's going on around you. In addition, exercise releases endorphins, which help you relax. Less helpful activities are passive ones like watching TV or spending too much time online. If you want to help speed up your recovery, look into the chapter on "Supercharge your Recovery."

If DP is particularly bad in the morning (as is most anxiety), try a cold shower to start your day. A few minutes in ice-cold water quickly remove any groggy feeling (a contributor to DP). Then dive straight into your day and keep yourself busy, all the while never pushing the DP away or getting too upset by it.

Try to remember each time you feel a wave of DP that this is a phase you're moving through, so be patient and kind to yourself while you're experiencing it. Adopt an attitude that all is well. Because it is. I know exactly how hard it is to keep your mind off DP because I've had firsthand experience with it myself, but these unusual sensations of depersonalization will always pass. Give it time. Once you've recovered from it, you'll find it hard to even remember what the state even felt like. If you want additional help speeding up your recovery from DP, study the chapter "Supercharge your Recovery."

As there is a strong element of disturbing/intrusive thoughts that go hand in hand with depersonalization, be sure to read the next section.

DISTURBING THOUGHTS

Anxiety almost always comes with a level of disturbing thoughts. You might be driving with your children and then get a flash thought of losing control and crashing into an oncoming car. Another example is looking down from a bridge and suddenly getting terrified by the idea that you might lose all control of your senses and jump.

If you experience such thoughts, I want to reassure you not to worry about them, regardless of how extreme they may be. They're the result of an anxious mind strained by exhaustion. They're not a signal that you're developing a neurotic illness. These thoughts persist because you react so strongly to them. If you didn't have a strong response, the thoughts would never bother you.

Disturbing thoughts occur to people who would never dream of doing the things they think about. It's the simple act of having the thoughts that shocks people and leads them to believe they're bad in some way. It's the anxious response to the thoughts that keeps them going around and around. I explain this in more detail in the chapter on giving up anxious thoughts.

For the moment, your best way to deal with this is to accept the chain of thoughts as they happen. When "terrible idea X" enters your mind, you can defuse it as follows:

"Oh whatever! I'm getting totally bored by all this fearmongering. It's not relevant to me or my life. But sure, go ahead, anxiety, and repeat that awful idea again if it makes you feel better."

Talk to the thoughts as if they're visitors that have no relationship to your real self; you're simply being polite by letting them run. Don't force them away—that creates the rebound effect. Instead, allow them to be but don't feel you have to pay them too much attention either. The goal is to move your attention back to what you were doing without responding in fear to the scary thought.

You know who you are and that these thoughts don't represent you, so don't worry. The very fact that you get so upset by the thoughts shows how different you are from the ideas that torment you. Another way to view the thoughts is as if they were school bullies trying to upset you by saying awful things about people close to you. If you get scared or annoyed, the bully continues to taunt you even more. If you laugh and say, *"Ummm, sure, anxiety, whatever,"* then walk away, the bully loses interest.

Acceptance and allowing are the keys here. What you really need to adopt is an attitude that all is well. Because it is. These fears are a nuisance, but they'll pass with the reduction of your general anxiety. Just hang in there. (I discuss disturbing thoughts in more detail in the chapter "Give Up Fearing Anxious Thoughts.")

DEPRESSION

Depression is a very large subject. I'll mention here only how it ties in with anxiety because that's the focus of this book. When someone has been feeling anxious for quite some time, the experience can become very frustrating and can lead to feeling depressed. Depression, in this context, is driven by thoughts of a future full of anxiety and restriction. A once carefree person now feels bound. In addition to having to cope with new restrictions, an anxiety disorder often comes with health fears, which contribute to further feelings of despair.

If you tackle the anxiety, you'll see a marked improvement in your overall sense of well-being. As your anxiety problem clears, the depressed state turns to one of hope. Hope is the antidote to depression. It gives you a reason to keep pursuing your goal of an anxiety-free life. Even though there's little scope here in this book to go into too much detail, The DARE Response can be equally applied to feelings of depression. Again, be mindful first of "what if" thoughts that surface and try to trap you in the stagnant energy of depression. A "whatever" mindset in response to them can be difficult to muster, but it's totally possible. Again, like the bully saying terrible things about you, you dismiss the thoughts as meaningless and untrue.

Allow the anxiety around depression to be present and mindfully sit with it without trying to force it away or beat yourself up for feeling this way. Once you feel ready, try to engage with something that keeps you from ruminating on how you're feeling. We really need an entire book on this subject, but the chapter on Give up Being So Hard on Yourself is very relevant for people who struggle with depression.

FEAR OF "GOING CRAZY"

I know some of you reading this fear that your anxiety might lead to a mental disorder like schizophrenia or bipolar disorder. It's understandable. Because there is so little public awareness of mental disease, people often jump to extreme conclusions. These conclusions are usually based on misinformation and an overactive imagination.

You need to understand that people don't "go crazy" in a sudden or spontaneous way. Major mental disorders like schizophrenia or bipolar disorder generally begin very gradually, not suddenly (such as during a panic attack). Stress or anxiety doesn't cause the disorder.

A further important point is that people who become schizophrenic have usually shown some mild symptoms (unusual thoughts, flowery speech, etc.) for most of their lives. Thus, if this hasn't been noticed yet in you, then chances are you won't become schizophrenic. This is especially true if you're over twenty-five since schizophrenia generally first appears in the late teens to early twenties.

CONCLUSION

I want to emphasize how important it is to let go of trying to control every anxious sensation you feel. Your body has an innate intelligence for keeping you alive and functioning perfectly. The less your conscious mind tries to interfere with that the better.

If you find yourself getting too anxious about any anxious thought or bodily sensation, apply The DARE Response and then let go.

Learn to let go and let your body do what it does best. Think of all the years your body has managed perfectly without your anxious mind's input. You must learn to surrender and trust again.

So, let go and trust your heart. Let go and trust your chest. Let go and trust your mind. Let go and trust whatever the sensation is that's scaring you.

Here's a summary of how to apply The DARE Response to any anxious physical or mental sensation.

- As a sensation manifests, immediately **defuse** the initial anxiety with a "so what" or "whatever" response.

- **Allow** each and every sensation to be. Get comfortable with the anxious sensations. Accept them as they are and don't resist them or force them away. If they morph into something else, allow that too.

- If the sensation is increasing and causing you a sense of threat, **run toward** it. Get excited and demand more of that sensation. Call out for it to get even more intense. Bring it on! This paradoxical request stops the escalation of fear.

- Lastly, **engage** your mind with an activity in the moment that grabs your full attention. Try your very best not to keep checking in on your anxiety to see if it's still there.

TIP: The Internet is a wonderful source of information, but the worst thing you can do is to try to self-diagnose yourself online. If you have a recurring health worry about a particular sensation, then go back to your primary care physician and have them put your mind to rest about that sensation. That may mean getting more tests run. Sometimes it helps to have that extra reassurance of further tests to really put a health worry to bed, but once you get that reassurance, trust it and stop second-guessing it! There's a saying that anxiety is like a disease of uncertainty. Don't fall into the trap of letting your anxious mind doubt your own health, especially when everything else is telling you otherwise.

GIVE UP FEARING THESE SITUATIONS

"The cave you fear
to enter holds the
treasure you seek."

-Joseph Campbell

So how did you go from having nothing troubling you to being afraid to go shopping or sit and have your hair cut? You're smart and competent; you've traveled far and wide. So why is it that now you have to white-knuckle your way through everyday situations that never caused you anxiety before?

The answer is actually quite simple. You became afraid of anxious bodily sensations. That fear has rocked your confidence in your body's ability to handle itself in certain situations. It's never really the situation you have to handle—it's yourself.

This loss of confidence doesn't happen overnight. You didn't wake up one day suddenly unable to do all of these things that you fear now. It was a slow process of anxiety eroding your confidence bit by bit. Such fears can often be traced back to one incident. For example, maybe you were in a line and had an anxious sensation manifest. That experience was enough to scare you, and from that moment on, you started to avoid lines. Or maybe you were stuck in traffic and had your first panic attack. Your mind then makes the connection that driving is something to fear, so now you fear driving and begin to avoid it.

In this simple way, avoidance creeps in. When we initially avoid situations, we feel some relief, and that relief from discomfort reinforces our avoidance. The problem, however, is that avoidance is a trap—in fact, it's the death knell of freedom. Over time, avoidance turns a fear of a situation into a phobia of it. A phobia is defined as an extreme or irrational fear of or aversion to something.

People who suffer from anxiety may develop phobias about driving, flying, or being in enclosed spaces (with no easy exit) or crowded spaces. The list is really quite long. It can include fear of not having a safe person with you, fear of being anywhere out of your safe zone, etc. There's a clinical phobia term for almost every situation you can imagine.

It's easy to understand why phobias develop. It all ties back to a loss of confidence in the ability to tolerate anxious sensations. Because of this lack of confidence, an anxious person defaults to managing their anxiety by avoiding a particular situation at all costs.

Avoidance can work for a while, but eventually it traps you. It shrinks and restricts your life, depriving you of many things that could bring you joy. The typical progression of avoidance has three stages:

A. having a panic attack in a particular situation

B. associating the situation with danger

C. avoiding that situation whenever possible

It never ceases to amaze me how creative people can become when they want to avoid something. I'm talking about planning out each and every detail of their day so that they don't have to stray out of their comfort zone and face certain situations that makes them anxious. This comfort zone eventually becomes a prison. In order to break free of this prison, you need to step outside of it using The DARE Response.

THE "WHAT IFS" AND TRYING TO CONTROL SITUATIONS

In the examples that follow, I'm going to demonstrate how to apply The DARE Response in a variety of real-life situations. As it would require too much space to go through each and every situation, I'm going to instead give examples of the most common ones. If I don't cover a specific situation that you struggle with, you'll still get a very good understanding of how to handle it by reading the examples below.

Basically, every avoidance maneuver has two main components, the "what ifs" (which you're familiar with from other parts of this book) and trying to control situations.

The "what ifs" are really the driving force behind all situational anxiety.

What if I go shopping and get overwhelmed?

What if I get on the plane and the anxiety is too much for me to handle?

What if I lose control and do something humiliating in front of others I know?

"What ifs" are the sparks that ignite the flame of fear and anxiety in situations—if they're allowed to. In an effort to curtail the impact of the "what ifs," an anxious person will try to control situations.

If a person has to face a situation that they associate with panic and anxiety, they'll worry about it for days or even weeks in advance.

They may need the assistance of a crutch, such as a safe person or medication, to get them through it. When they do have to encounter such a situation, the anxious person will often prepare an "out."

Typical "outs" include:

- sitting on the outside of a row of seats for easy access to the exit

- pretending to get an important call if you feel the need to bail

- always driving your own car so that you never have to wait for a ride home or sit in the passenger seat of another person's vehicle

- always knowing where the toilet is in case you suddenly have to go or just need to be alone for a bit

- always having a phone close at hand in case you need to call for help

Trying to control situations in this manner is as unhelpful as avoiding them because you're still sending the message to yourself that you're in potential danger when, of course, you aren't. A panic attack isn't going to kill you. You're as perfectly safe on a deserted island with panic and anxiety as you are sitting in a hospital surrounded by doctors. So understand that physiologically you really aren't in any more danger at Walmart than you are at home. When you come to really understand this, you can see that all you have to master in the end is yourself—not the situation. The anxiety isn't in the situation; it's in your *response to the feelings* you have in the situation.

What you're going to learn below is how to develop a higher tolerance of anxious sensations in different situations. Learning to feel confident and safe in the situations that make you anxious is the secret to overcoming your fear. The DARE Response can be used in a variety of situations. **As in the previous chapter on sensations, you can skip ahead to the situation that is most applicable to you. But be sure and check back in again at the Conclusion to**

this chapter where more helpful tips and tricks for dealing with all of these situations are located.

The situations I'll discuss here are:

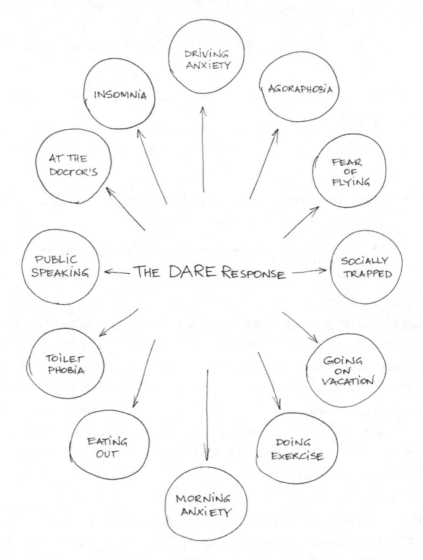

Let's begin by giving examples of how you might apply The DARE Response to situations where you feel there's no easy escape—driving, enclosed spaces, flying, and public speaking.

THE DARE RESPONSE FOR DRIVING ANXIETY

One of the more common questions I'm asked is how to apply The DARE Response while driving. People have many different fears in this area, ranging from fear of being caught in traffic to crossing waterway bridges. Often the anxiety stems from a fear of being trapped in the vehicle in gridlock traffic or losing control of the vehicle and causing a collision.

Needless to say, even though they may have been battling a driving phobia for many years, almost all the people I've consulted with have not actually had any of these mishaps occur. Let's look at the primary fear: having an accident due to the distractions of an anxiety attack while driving.

Most people work themselves into a state of high anxiety even before they've pulled out of their driveways. They imagine causing ten-car collisions on the highway because they "freaked out" and hit another vehicle. If you have such concerns, the first thing to do is review your driving history. Have you been a reckless driver in the past? Do you have a history of bad driving? Most phobic drivers actually have clean driving records and have never even been in a minor road incident. Anxious drivers are not a deadly hazard on the road; in fact, they can be a lot more vigilant than many ordinary drivers who, after a long day at the office, are virtually asleep at the wheel.

As we discussed previously, when looking at the biology of anxiety, by virtue of their conditions, anxious drivers have a high level of sensory alertness. This level of alertness keeps them aware of potential hazards and focused on the task of driving—they're not daydreaming, chatting, or rooting around in the glove compartment. This, of course, doesn't suggest that anxious driving is the ideal way to commute. But I believe it's important to make this point because so many people chastise themselves for being anxious in their cars. If you're generally a good driver, before you set out in your car, you can acknowledge and reaffirm that you're a capable driver. This should go some part of the way toward alleviating your concerns.

The second major concern of most phobic drivers is the fear of being trapped in their car in some manner. By this, I mean being caught in traffic, on busy three-lane highways, on long bridges, or even stopped at red lights. When allowed to, their mind will run away with this fear and imagine all kinds of deadly scenarios where they feel cornered or trapped in their vehicle with no assistance available should they experience a major panic attack.

The important thing here is to curb these "what if" fears before they take root by offering yourself viable solutions to any of these scenarios and not letting your mind trick you into believing there's a trap ahead. Give it some thought. Are there really any situations, such as the ones described above, where you're truly trapped with no means of escape?

No, of course there aren't.

Eventually, traffic always moves; it doesn't remain gridlocked forever. There's flow, and there's always an exit. This may mean figuring out the exit for yourself, but never let these thoughts corner you into thinking there's no escape. When you counteract these fears with logical solutions, you undermine the control that fear holds over you.

I'm going to show you how to apply The DARE Response to driving anxiety. I suggest that you begin by taking your car out on a practice run, possibly at night or on a Sunday when there's less traffic. Drive a route that you feel anxious about; perhaps go beyond your safety zone or drive over a bridge. If you feel very nervous, begin with a smaller test. The important thing, though, is to challenge yourself with a route that causes you at least some degree of concern. You won't be long into the journey before the anxiety starts to manifest itself. This anxiety may be low level, but if driving really is a problem, it will gradually manifest itself into feelings of panic or anxiety.

As you feel that panic rise and "what if" fears manifesting, begin by **defusing** each of those fears with a confident, dismissive response. For example:

What if I have a panic attack in the car far from home?

So what! I have the tools to get through it now. I know I can handle it.

What if the car breaks down and I get stuck all alone?

So what! I'll just call for help. It won't be long before someone comes to help me.

What if I get anxious crossing a bridge or driving through a tunnel?

Whatever! The wave of panic will pass as soon as I use The DARE Response. I've been through much worse.

What if I feel too dizzy and can't drive?

Whatever! I'll find a safe place to pull over and take a break until it passes.

Defuse these "what ifs" quickly and allow the nervous arousal you feel to just be there with you as you drive. Tell yourself you're going to **allow it** to manifest whatever way it wishes. You're going to be totally comfortable with whatever anxious discomfort you feel in the car. Say to yourself as you drive: "*I accept and allow these anxious feelings. I accept and allow these anxious thoughts.*"

As you accept and allow, it's natural that "what if" thoughts will continue to pop into your mind. They're to be expected. If they grab your attention, be sure to answer them with a dismissive "so what" or "whatever."

If you feel the bodily sensations of nervous arousal increasing into a rush of adrenaline (a panic attack), **run toward** your fear. Tell yourself how excited you feel to be driving and demand that your anxiety make your sensations more intense.

Tell your anxiety to bring it on and deliver a full-blown panic attack. Really demand it and get angry if you like. If you really demand more, the adrenaline flood will stop quickly, and you'll return to a much lower level of nervous arousal that you can allow to be fully present.

If you feel safer pulling over to do this, then please do so. If you do feel lightheaded and faint, pull over and continue with The DARE Response in a parked position. We don't want you too distracted while driving, but it's possible for many people to still complete this step even while driving. You know your own self best, so do whatever you're most comfortable with. If you do keep driving, the important thing is to keep focused on the road and drive at a safe speed.

Finally, **engage** fully with your driving. Pay attention to everything that's going on around you. Pay attention to all the other vehicles around you. If you find that your mind keeps wandering back to anxious "what if" fears, you might want to turn on some music and start singing.

The car, after the shower, is the next best place to sing out loud. Singing is a great release of pent-up nervous energy around your throat and chest area, so put on your favorite tune and belt one out! It really does help release nervous energy.

When you take your car on a test run, you should be aware that you're going to feel anxious discomfort. If there's no anxiety manifesting, then maybe you're not pushing out of your comfort zone enough. The real learning happens and real confidence is built when you feel anxious yet still complete the task. The initial goal is *not* to eliminate your anxious sensations; it's to drive with them regardless of whether they're present or not.

These practice drives can be done with another person the first few times to help build up your confidence. If you don't have someone to practice with, hire a driving instructor to do it with you. After more practice, I recommend then driving alone—that's when you develop true independence and freedom from fear. If you always practice with another individual, you may form the idea that it's your passenger who's helping you feel safe and that can hold your progress back. If you find it hard to drive on busy roads, then practice during times of the day when there's little to no traffic (e.g., very early on Sunday mornings).

"Wherever you go, there you are." - Buddha

It's very common for a person with driving anxiety to fear passing a certain distance away from their safe zone (usually their home). The anxious "what if" thought is: *"What if I go too far and have a panic attack and can't get back?"* This fear applies to all travel away from home.

What you have to understand is that distance is really irrelevant. How far you go isn't important. What is important is how you handle each and every wave of anxiety that manifests. This is a physiological issue going on within your own mind and body, and it doesn't matter whether you're sitting on your front porch or aboard the space station. It's always about your response, so don't focus on the distance; focus on your response.

I appreciate, however, that in the beginning you still have to prove this to yourself with experience, so if driving a certain distance from home is a concern, then break it down into smaller steps. Start by determining what your safe zone in your mind is and then begin by pushing yourself to drive just outside that safe zone. That might be five, ten, or fifty miles from your home. When you get there, part of you'll feel like "Great! I did it. Now let's rush back home in case something happens." Instead, I want you to just stop the car and *stay there a while*. Stay there seated in your car until you get a bit bored. This is very important to do because it means you're pushing the boundary out and keeping it out. You own that new distance, your world has gotten that much bigger, and so has your confidence. Now you start to appreciate that the distance you go is really an illusion. The only thing that matters is how you respond to the waves of anxiety wherever you find yourself. (See more on this in the sections below, Agoraphobia and Going on Holidays.)

The DARE Response will give you the ability to move into the fear of any road situation. Moving with your anxious discomfort while driving brings your confidence back.

THE DARE RESPONSE FOR SOCIALLY TRAPPED SITUATIONS

By "socially trapped" situations, I mean any situation in which you might find yourself where you feel you can't easily leave or excuse yourself from it because of some kind of social embarrassment.

Typical examples might be:

- getting your hair cut

- standing in line while shopping

- sitting in a work meeting

- sitting in a row of seats (e.g., the cinema or church)

- eating out in a restaurant

- sitting in the passenger seat of someone's car

- riding an elevator

All of these situations have similar "what if" thoughts about feeling trapped and the social embarrassment that might follow. The first thing you must remember is that you're not really "trapped" in any of these situations. There is no one holding you there against your will. Your sense of being trapped has more to do with your fear of what others might think if you decide to suddenly excuse yourself. **Defuse** those "what if" thoughts as they arise, like this:

"What if I start to panic and need to leave my shopping behind?"

So what? If I really need to, I'll just walk out the door—simple.

"What will these people think of me if I walk out?"

So what? I'll make an excuse and go. "Hey, got to run. Sorry folks, bye."

"What if it's too awkward or difficult to leave?"

So what if it's awkward? If I want to go, I'll go. I'm nobody's prisoner.

So what if it means upsetting a few people? They're adults. I'm sure they'll get over it.

Remember, you're not answering these "what ifs" in order to come up with a plan of avoidance; you're answering them so that they don't spark more anxiety and trap you into an ever-increasing cycle of fear.

I'm going to use "getting a haircut" as an example below, but what I describe applies to almost any situation where you fear not being able to escape easily.

Before you go to get your hair cut, acknowledge to yourself that you're most likely going to feel anxious. Fully expect the anxiety so that when it does show up, it doesn't catch you off guard.

As you relax into the salon chair and begin to make small talk, you'll feel your anxiety peak a little bit. It may be a bodily tension or some other uncomfortable sensation. As the anxiety rises, so too will the "what if" fears, so immediately **defuse** them:

"What if I need to leave halfway through?"

So what? I'll make an excuse and tell them I'll be back shortly. No big deal. This happens all the time.

You then start to **allow** all that nervous energy to just be there with you as you get your hair cut. Invite it to sit with you. Remind yourself that for the next little while as you're getting your hair cut, you're going to be totally okay with *any* anxious discomfort you feel. Allow it all. Say to yourself, "I accept and allow these anxious feelings. I accept and allow these anxious thoughts."

There may come a point—usually only a few minutes after sitting down—where your anxiety can spike and you feel a sudden rush of adrenaline. Normally, this would scare you and be an indicator of a panic attack coming on, but not anymore because now you know what to do.

You **run toward** it. You get excited and demand more. You turn that fear of panic into a rush of excitement and demand that your anxiety make the sensation you feel more intense. Your mind might keep flashing with "what ifs," but they get canceled out by the very fact that you're demanding more. You know this is all just a flood of adrenaline and it will pass. In fact, you're so familiar and comfortable with this rush that you demand even more of it just to see what happens. You're in a playful, excited mood; you're not panicked.

Do this with real commitment, and the adrenaline flood will quickly pass, leaving you with the same nervous, jittery feeling you had when you first sat in the chair.

Finally, start to **engage** with something. You could read a magazine, but it's even better to engage in conversation with the person cutting your hair. Conversations are always better as they require more of your attention, plus they trigger a social connection, which has a positive mood-enhancing effect.

You're then back to allowing the nervous arousal to just be with you and talking about where you're thinking of going on your next vacation.

The above is an example that can be applied to almost every situation from which you feel you can't easily excuse yourself (e.g., getting your hair cut, attending a show, or sitting in a work meeting).

It's really important to work through your anxiety in the situation as best you can. If you leave early because of the anxiety, you'll feel defeated, as if the anxiety has the upper hand.

But what about situations where there is absolutely no exit?

THE DARE RESPONSE FOR FEAR OF FLYING AND PHYSICALLY TRAPPED SITUATIONS

Flying is good example of a situation that you can't leave (once the plane is on its way). You can apply this same advice to any situation where you're really not able to get physically out of the situation (e.g., in an elevator, having a full body scan, or at the dentist).

Before I describe The DARE Response for a fear of flying, I want to point out that this is designed for the fear of having a panic attack or high anxiety while flying because there is no escape. If your fear relates to a fear of the plane crashing due to some mechanical failure, I recommend a course like Capt. Tom Bunn's SOAR program, which teaches you just how safe flying is.

"What if" thoughts are the main fuel (pardon the pun!) that power a fear of flying. So let's examine them: What is really the worst that can happen?

You know already that a panic attack won't kill you. You're not going to suffocate, and fainting from anxiety is very rare. You also know that the overwhelming majority of people who have full-blown panic attacks do so without people around even noticing. They don't lose control or act out in an impulsive or dangerous manner. So the worst that really will happen is that you'll feel very uncomfortable for a period of time on an airplane.

Unpleasant, yes—but not life-threatening.

When you keep that in mind, being in a situation like flying in an airplane doesn't seem such an awful prospect. You'll get through it. But that was before you read this book. Now you have the tools to make that unpleasant experience more pleasant—to the point where you might actually even enjoy the flight.

I'm going to demonstrate how to apply The DARE Response for fear of flying so that you can feel confident and safe while flying both long and short distances.

A good flight starts the night before. Try to ensure that you get some good rest before your departure. Fatigue can cause excess stress. On the day of the flight, organize your schedule as best as possible, ensuring that there is no hassle getting to the airport, passing through security, etc. You can do this by giving yourself plenty of time. There's no point in adding more stress to an already nervous trip simply because you have to rush through the airport at the last minute.

As you board the plane, *don't hope that you'll feel relaxed and calm.* Instead, expect that you most likely *will* experience anxiety.

Now take your seat and reframe the anxious feelings you have by telling yourself over and over:

"I'm excited to be flying. I'm excited to be flying."

And so you should be. Flying is exciting. Allow your body to express that excitement.

Remember, "what if" thoughts are guaranteed. **Defuse** each and every one of them that tugs at you.

"What if the anxiety gets really bad and I have nowhere to run?"

So what! If it gets really bad, yes, it will be uncomfortable, but it won't kill me. It will pass. It can't keep escalating.

"What if we experience bad turbulence?"

Whatever! I'll treat it like an exciting rollercoaster ride. I know I'm safe and that airplanes can easily handle the very worst turbulence.

As you settle in, **allow** all the nervous arousal you feel to be there with you. Let it accompany you on this journey. Invite it to stay, and tell it that you know it will probably get more intense during takeoff and in moments of turbulence—but that's okay, too. Repeat over and over to yourself: "I accept and allow this anxious feeling. I accept and allow these anxious thoughts."

If at any point during the flight you feel that familiar flood of adrenaline and think you might be about to have a panic attack, respond with the following:

"There you are. I was expecting you to show up at some point on this flight."

You were never trying to run away from it; in fact, you were hoping it would emerge so that you could **run toward** it.

"Well, let's get to it!" Then demand to experience more of the anxious sensations that you feel. I know this is hard to do when in an enclosed situation like an airplane, but trust me—it's the right response.

The more you really get excited and demand to have a panic attack during the flight, the more empowered and confident you'll feel in yourself because you're placing yourself in a position of power. It can sometimes help to become a bit emotional with the fear when you demand it to show itself because this helps the emotions to release and flow.

Expect a rush of adrenaline on takeoff; this is usually the most anxious moment of the flight for people. Notice how the adrenaline has that wavelike effect. It courses through your body—and if you pay close attention, you'll feel it pass quickly, in twenty or thirty seconds. Nothing to fear here. After it passes, confidence returns— until the next wave comes, and the next, until eventually you notice the pattern. And, by not responding in fear, the effect on you is nothing more than bodily sensations minus the fear and panic.

Once the feeling of heightened anxiety has subsided, place your full attention on something. **Engage** with a pleasurable activity that interests you. That might mean reading a magazine or watching some in-flight entertainment. If you have relaxing music, now is a good time to play it.

You'll probably find it hard to sleep during the flight, but do try to relax into it as much as possible. Maybe you'll even enjoy it!

I recommend you bring an eye mask for longer flights as well as some relaxing music to play so that you can retreat into your own relaxed space and are not distracted by people around you. Better yet, download my free audio to help you relax during the flight here:

visit www.DareResponse.com/app

THE DARE RESPONSE FOR FEAR OF PUBLIC SPEAKING

A really common question I get is: How do you implement The DARE Response when you don't have time to think? The short answer is that you use a modified version of The DARE Response.

The best way to illustrate that is to discuss public speaking as it combines a highly pressurized situation with the need to perform a task.

These speaking engagements don't necessarily have to be the traditional "on a podium" events; they can be as simple as an office meeting where you're expected to express an opinion or give verbal feedback. The fear is centered around being incapacitated by the anxiety and thus being unable to complete what you're saying. I've worked with everyone from TV presenters and famous entertainers to first-time public speakers—the approach is always one and the same.

As with all the situations treated in this chapter, preparation beforehand is key. I don't mean just the standard advice of preparing your material; I mean preparing the right mindset.

First of all, you should have a few responses prepared to help **defuse** the "what ifs" that might have you fleeing the spotlight with an undignified departure (or jumping out the office window):

"What if people notice I'm nervous?"

So what? I allow myself to be nervous so that I can present with an excited energy that engages the audience. I let my nerves show that I care about the subject I'm presenting.

"What if the anxiety is too much before I start?"

So what? I'm actually hoping to be anxious so that I can use that nervous energy to present better.

Accepting that you're going to be anxious before and during the speech is important. If you allow for that, it doesn't throw you just before you're about to begin. Once you begin talking, the real secret is to stop trying to be calm and composed. That mental effort is what causes you to spiral down into ever-increasing anxiety during a presentation. If, on the other hand, you give yourself permission to experience these anxious sensations, then it feels like everything is going exactly as it should. This is what happens when you **allow** yourself to be anxious. If that means you feel your throat tighten up, your heart pound wildly, or your voice crack during the speech— let it be so. Most of the top speakers in the world are riddled with anxiety before an event, but they always use this nervousness to enhance their speech or performance.

When you channel your nervous discomfort into the presentation, all your energies are going in the one same direction, instead of part of you trying hard to be calm and composed. No one wants calm and composed. People want to hear presenters who are alive and present. It's okay to let the world see you're nervous. That's more authentic, and it brings you very much into the moment, as opposed to being a speaker who appears totally bored and as if she or he has given this same presentation a hundred times before.

By channeling the nervous energy into the moment and allowing it to manifest, you're then moving in the same direction as the anxiety. Instead of pushing the emotional energy and excitement down into your stomach, you're expressing it out, discharging it. You can push it out even more by expressing yourself more forcefully or by being more animated, by moving around on stage. In this way, you allow the nervous energy to be released faster, and you'll feel alive and present very quickly. Actors always remark that stage fright ends the moment they begin; that's because they're doing exactly this.

They're expressing themselves in the moment. Yes, they have a slight advantage in that they're really performing and exaggerating their self-expression, but you can do the same in a more toned-down manner for any type of public-speaking engagement, be it addressing a somber business crowd or giving an emotional best man's speech.

If at any point before or even during your talk you feel your anxiety spike into a panic attack where your bodily sensations are getting very intense, then **run toward** it. Get more excited and demand more of it. Demanding more is a split-second thought you can fire off even between sentences. It's more of an attitude than anything else where you're standing up to your fear and saying, "Bring it on! Yes, even here and now. I can handle it." No matter how tough it gets, you'll always finish your piece—even if there are moments you feel you can't go on, keep pushing through.

You'll be surprised how quickly this simple step can slow your heart rate and stop the adrenaline flood. It gives you an immediate sense of power and control. When you notice the anxiety drop, fire off another quick thought and demand for it to come back. You demand more of the intense sensations because you're absolutely not threatened by them.

If you apply this approach, you'll give a great presentation as you'll come across alive, fully engaged, and present.

But how do you do all of this while speaking at the same time?

All of this is done in a split second. There's always a moment to do this on stage. You'd be amazed at how many different, unrelated thoughts you can have while speaking in front of people. In fact, you probably already have many unrelated thoughts when presenting. For example: *Are people reacting well to me? Why is that guy playing with his phone and not paying attention? Where's that person going?* Instead, I'm teaching you how to have empowering thoughts that will aid your presentation skills.

But what about the most dreaded "what if" of public speaking—forgetting what you need to say? Being present in the moment (with your anxiety) aids mental recall. If you're working off bullet-point notes, you'll find that you flow easily from one point to the next. The reason your recall is greatly improved is that your anxious mind is not getting in the way, trying to get rid of the anxiety you feel. So the recall from your short- and long-term memory is uninterrupted.

The additional bonus of being very present and engaged like this is that you'll also have the unique ability to respond to any interruption that happens in the room, e.g., an out-of-the-blue question or even a humorous heckle.

I want to point out however that I don't always get it right in this area. I too have the odd setback and sometimes forget to heed my own advice. So let me tell you a story about what *not to do* when performing in public…

Since liberating myself from anxiety, I've always looked for ways to challenge myself and to keep pushing outside my safe zone. A few years ago I did something I never dreamt I would do in the throes of anxiety and joined an amateur acting group. With acting not only is there the mortification of forgetting your lines, there's also a chance that you'll let the other actors down. Not to mention the director, the stage manager, the lighting guy…ahhh!

Our first production was a series of short plays on the theme of *Romance*. I was cast with an attractive young woman called Robin, who was also new to acting. Our scene together was that of a nervous first dinner date. We had rehearsed the scene a thousand times and both of us were very confident as we sat backstage, waiting to go on. In fact we were so confident that we thought it would be a good idea to start celebrating already and open the bottle of wine that was one of our props for the dinner scene. Our justification being that the scene was post dinner so we were only feeding our imaginations. We had a few glasses (or should I say I had a few glasses) and then topped the almost empty bottle up with water – who would know, right?

When it came time to go on stage I was feeling super confident and looking forward to my first time on stage in front of a packed theatre. We walked out on stage and sat down at the table, the lights came up and I had a complete blank! It was like the part of my brain where all my lines were stored was completely inaccessible. I am sure you are familiar with this feeling. You know the information is there and you have accessed it a thousand times before but for some reason you just can't get at it, it's like the file has been deleted.

Robin began the scene and luckily her first few lines triggered my first line by automatic response but then as she spoke again, I felt the sense of terror creep over me that I was going to inevitably forget my lines at some point.

What was interesting was that the scene was supposed to be a very awkward first date and I had stopped acting and was genuinely feeling very awkward. The cool calm from backstage was gone and the anxiety of making a total fool of myself was ever present. Then of course it happened. It was my turn to speak and I had no idea what to say. I drew a complete blank. I had no option but to call for my line by shouting out 'line' to the assistant director who was offstage. Now my self-confidence was shot and I was feeling totally self-conscious just wishing the scene would come to an end. I muddled through the rest of the scene and when we got off stage I swore to myself that I would never have a drink before a play again.

Ironically, the director said it was probably the best scene of the night because the audience thought our genuine discomfort was down to innate talent. If only my fellow acting partner had felt that way, we never saw her again.

Since then we have done several plays all of which have been a real pleasure to participate in but that first episode really made me acutely aware of how alcohol can have a disastrous effect when performing in public. You might think it's a good idea: that it will help calm your nerves before a presentation or performance but, you have been warned, it can have a dramatic effect on your memory recall. Small amounts before a Best Man speech is fine but other than that it's a crutch – a rubber one!

THE DARE RESPONSE TO END AGORAPHOBIA

Agoraphobia is defined as an extreme or irrational fear of open or public places. What that really translates into is an extreme fear of having a panic attack anywhere outside the home. I think a lot of people who have regular panic attacks experience some degree of agoraphobia. Some of them might call themselves *functioning agoraphobics*, meaning they can function within a small radius of their home—they can shop locally or maybe pick the kids up from school, but they can't do much outside that zone.

The agoraphobic person fears that if a panic attack does occur, who would look after them and how would they get assistance and reassurance? They feel at the mercy of the place in which they find themselves and the strangers around them. In its extreme form, agoraphobia can lead to a situation where people become totally housebound for long periods of time.

If you're agoraphobic, please see the chapter "Give up Your Safe Zone" for advice on how to push outside your safe zone using The DARE Response.

THE DARE RESPONSE GOING ON VACATION

It's appropriate to briefly mention a really common fear, which is the fear of going on vacation. This kind of situation usually raises the following fears

-getting upset at the idea of being far from home

-feeling uncomfortable in strange, new surroundings (e.g., strange food, sights/sounds)

-fear of vacationing with people (friends/in-laws) who might not understand your problem

-fear of being unable to enjoy it and spending every minute wishing to be back home again

Taking a vacation is a great way to build confidence as it gives you an opportunity to really step outside your safe zone, have new opportunities to practice The DARE Response, and build your confidence up. Your confidence will soar because you'll really grasp the idea that distance is irrelevant. It's always about you and how you're handling the anxiety as it manifests, regardless of where you're located.

Armed with The DARE Response, you can now go on vacation confident that whatever happens, you'll be able to handle it.

The hardest part is actually the anticipation of the vacation—worrying about the flight, worrying about the accommodation, worrying about getting home. Worrying like that is to be expected before a vacation, especially if it's something you haven't done in a long time. Use The DARE Response to defuse this anticipatory anxiety as well, and trust me that once you actually begin your vacation, your anxiety won't be the problem you fear it will be. The added bonus of being on vacation is that you get absorbed by the new surroundings and activities and, as a result, spend less time ruminating over your anxiety. If anxiety does manifest on your vacations, don't start to get upset. Simply understand that this was never about not being anxious on your vacations; it's about being able to still enjoy yourself and be there with your friends and family regardless of anxiety or not. That's a huge achievement. You go with the mindset of bringing your anxiety with you on vacation—pack a little bag for it. If it stays the whole trip, well and good. The important thing is that you don't let it stop you from going.

When you get back home, your confidence will soar because you'll have really proved to yourself that the idea of a safe zone is an illusion. You traveled well outside your safe zone and even ended up having a good time. Now challenges at home seem all the more manageable.

THE DARE RESPONSE FOR MORNING ANXIETY

Many people with anxiety will report that mornings are the hardest. You may be interested to know that there is scientific evidence to explain why. The vast majority of people experience higher levels of the stress hormone cortisol in the morning. For some, there can be an increase of about 50 percent in cortisol levels occurring twenty to thirty minutes *after* awakening in the morning. Following this, cortisol levels decline throughout the day, with the lowest levels occurring during the first half of the night.

This raised level of cortisol is felt more acutely by those that are highly anxious and sensitized already. Compounding all of this is the sluggish nature of our body and mind in the morning, which can create a haze-like effect, leading to more frustration and worry. We have the expression, *"He/she is not a morning person."* It's the reason why people drink coffee every morning—to snap out of this morning haze.

For this reason it's important to be mindful of what's happening in your body and not to get upset by it. It doesn't mean that you aren't making progress or that your anxiety is getting worse. It will lift as the morning moves on, especially if you apply The DARE Response. Allow the anxiety to be, and channel the nervous energy you feel into positive action! Now take the following, additional steps:

1. Drink a large glass of **fresh water**.

2. Open the window for some fresh air, and then begin some **light stretching**.

3. Next take a **cold shower!** No, it's not particularly pleasant, but you'll feel mentally much more alert as the anxious haze lifts with the shock of the cold water. If that's too intense for you, then vary the temperature between cold and warm. There are health benefits to a cold shower too. Studies show our body's

immune system benefits because the number of white blood cells produced increases when we take regular cold showers.

4. Eat a **good breakfast**. Be sure to avoid refined sugar, coffee, and caffeinated teas. Instead, have a cup of hot water with a slice of lemon. This is a really great way to give your whole system (in particular, your liver) a healthy morning boost. Never skip breakfast, no matter how pushed for time you are.

5. If you don't have something in particular to do each morning, then you must find something to do. **Don't hang around.** If you're idle, your mind will turn inwards and go back to "checking in" on your anxiety. What you want is to be busy from the get-go and have a purpose to your morning. The distraction of having something purposeful to do is often the key to moving you out of anxious feelings faster.

THE DARE RESPONSE FOR INSOMNIA AND NIGHT PANIC

The two things that keep people awake at night are physical pain and/or worry. Insomnia is defined as habitual sleeplessness. When it manifests, it develops into a worry of not being able to sleep that can play on a person's mind hours before they actually have to go bed. It's a vicious cycle.

To break the cycle of insomnia, you have to be allowing of whatever happens at night. Don't try to force sleep as that will only add to the problem. You approach each night as simply a possible opportunity to sleep. By doing this, you remove the pressure you're placing yourself under. Here is how to apply The DARE Response in this situation.

In a way, some people have performance anxiety when they think about sleeping. They ask themselves: *Will I be able to make myself sleep tonight?*

The answer is maybe yes, maybe no. If you're going through a period of sleeplessness, a good night's sleep isn't guaranteed, for whatever reason, so you have to accept that for the moment. **Defuse** those anxious "what ifs" with a dismissive statement like:

"Whatever. If I get one or two hours of sleep, that's well and good, and if I don't sleep at all, I'll survive."

Then **allow** whatever is going to happen that night to happen. This open acceptance will transform the frustration you feel regarding not being able to sleep. Each night, as you go to bed, say to yourself:

I'm preparing for bed, but I won't try to force sleep.

If it comes, it comes. If not, I won't beat myself up over it.

This is a period I'm going through, but I'll soon return to normal sleep patterns.

It's natural for every person to go through periods of sleeplessness from time to time. After a certain point, however, the anger and frustration of not sleeping is what keeps you awake, so let me emphasize again the importance of accepting your temporary inability to sleep. Surrender to whatever may or may not happen during the course of a night, and you'll put your mind under much less pressure.

If you really find yourself wrestling with the frustration of not sleeping, then **run toward** that and try to stay awake instead. Tell yourself that you are going to try your best to remain awake the entire night. This alone can be enough to end the frustration and allow you to doze off soon after.

Avoid **engaging** with your "to-do" list or replaying any negative events of the day in your mind; instead, just focus on your breath as you lie in bed.

Here are some additional tips on how to create the most advantageous conditions for sleep and also what you can do when you simply can't nod off.

- If possible have a warm bath with several drops of lavender oil before bed. Your muscles will start to relax in the warm water, and the smell of the lavender oil triggers a calming response. Hot water releases muscle tension and reduces restlessness, making it easier for you to relax into a bed. If you can't take a bath, then have a long, hot shower.

- Take 300mg of magnesium before going to bed. Magnesium is a great sleep aid as it helps with muscle relaxation. (More on magnesium in the Supercharge your Recovery chapter)

- Set the right temperature for you room. If you're in a cooler room rather than one that's too warm, it's easier for sleep to happen. The recommended temperature is between 65 and 72 degrees Fahrenheit (18 to 22 Celsius), but you may need to play around with that to find your ideal temperature. For the majority of people, having the room too warm or using too many blankets is a major cause of restless sleep patterns.

- If your mind is very active, read fiction for a short period in bed before turning off the light. Fiction is a mental-state changer. It stimulates the right side of your brain, which is the side that controls imagination and visualization, and it helps to turn off the analytical brain, which loves to worry about tomorrow. Be sure the book is something light— nothing too gripping or you might never put it down. It needs to be fiction (not newspapers or business books) for this to be effective because fiction allows you to escape your daily thought patterns.

- Use an eye mask. People with anxiety tend to be quite sensitive to light and sound. Even the slightest light entering the room may be hindering your ability to sleep. The added advantage with the eye mask is that if you wake early in the morning and the room is getting brighter, you won't be affected by this with the mask on. It takes only about three nights of using an eye mask to get accustomed to it.

- If you wake in the middle of the night, don't leave your bed—try to stay there. Getting up takes you farther out of the sleep pattern. It's best if you stay in bed lying down with the light off because that sends a message to your brain that it really is bedtime. If you're very awake, try reading some more fiction and then turn off the light as soon as you feel sleepy again.

- Should you find your mind racing and you simply can't stop obsessing about a certain matter, turn the light on, get a pen and paper, and start writing your worries down (e.g., "Tomorrow I have to do X, Y, Z and I'm afraid I won't be well rested," and "What if …," etc.). Continue to write down your worries until the exercise becomes tedious. It's important to overdo it so that your mind releases the mental energy keeping you awake onto paper. Often one of the reasons we can't fall asleep is that our mind feels these worries are important to analyze over and over. Writing down all your worries has the effect of saying to your mind: "Okay, mind, you think these are important. I've written them all down in detail. They won't be forgotten, I promise. I can come back to them tomorrow and deal with them then—but RIGHT NOW, let's sleep." The mind can be like a small child who just needs reassurance that things will be dealt with and looked after. That's all it needs to let go of these mental worries. You then discover, in the morning, that almost all the worries or concerns aren't big issues.

NIGHT PANIC

People with anxiety disorders can sometimes be awakened at night by panic attacks. Some describe it like this:

"Just as I'm about to drop off to sleep, my body seems to jolt awake, like an electric shock, which then frightens me and keeps me awake for hours."

This jolt is called a hypnic jerk, or hypnagogic massive jerk. A hypnic jerk usually occurs just as the person enters sleep. People often describe it as a falling sensation or an electric shock, and it's a completely normal experience. It's most common when we're sleeping uncomfortably or when we're overtired. There's been little research on the subject, but there are some theories as to why hypnic jerks occur. When we drift off into sleep, the body undergoes changes in temperature, breathing, and muscle relaxation. The hypnic jerk may be a result of the muscles relaxing. The brain misinterprets this as a sign of falling, and it signals our limbs to wake up, hence the jerking legs or arms.

People turn hypnic jerks into panic attacks because they already feel nervous about their condition, and the jolt scares them into thinking something bad is happening. Again, it's a fearful response to a sensation. Usually when these people jolt awake, they get a fright and gasp for air, which can then turn into the fear of a breathing or heart problem while sleeping.

If you wake like this, then simply understanding the nature of a hypnic jerk can strip the anxiety away from the experience. Reassure yourself that you're safe and that the jerk isn't something to worry about. It doesn't disrupt your bodily functions, and it doesn't put you in any danger. As a side point, people who have a fear of flying often experience this jolt on long-haul flights because they drift off to sleep in an uncomfortable position and then suddenly jolt awake. Jolting awake like this causes them more anxiety because they're on an airplane.

THE DARE RESPONSE FOR ANXIETY EXERCISING/IN THE GYM

One of the biggest triggers for people who have panic attacks is to experience an intense bodily sensation out of the blue as it were. Sensations like a pounding heart, increased respiration, or hot flashes (which we detailed in the previous chapter) can be very unsettling, and yet these are exactly the sensations created from vigorous workouts. This is why many people report having panic attacks in the gym and develop a phobia around doing any exercise that might recreate these sensations.

Armed with The DARE Response, workouts are now going to become your new way of building your confidence in your body back up. What follows is a strategy for anyone who has a fear of intense bodily sensations (which pretty much includes everyone who has panic attacks).

The aim is to go to the park or gym and work out with the sole intention of getting comfortable with aroused bodily sensations. I'm going to use the treadmill as an example, but this can be applied to any workout that increases your heart rate and causes you to sweat.

Start with a brisk walk and then work up to a low- to medium-paced jog on the treadmill. As soon as the sensations (pounding heart, sweating, increased respiration) are present, slow back down to a brisk walk. Now, as you walk, practice The DARE Response with the sensations that are still present. **Defuse** anxious "what if" thinking.

"What if my heart won't stop pounding?"

"Whatever, if it keeps pounding, let it."

"What if my breathing stays so labored?"

"Oh well, if it does, that's fine. No big deal. It will eventually settle down."

Allow all sensations to be present. Repeat over and over to yourself: "I accept and allow this anxious feeling. I accept and allow these anxious thoughts."

If you feel the anxiety is escalating into a sense of panic, **run toward it.** Demand more. You can demand more by requesting that your heart pound even faster or that your breathing get even more intense.

The good thing about walking and not running at this stage is that you know in the back of your mind that the sensations are decreasing anyway as your body is calming down from an exerted state.

After a few minutes, all the sensations will have disappeared and your body will be in a comfortable state just walking on the treadmill. When you're ready, pick up the pace again to a jog and repeat the procedure. What you're really looking to do here is to stimulate the sensations just enough so that they're present, but not too much so that they overwhelm you. You're giving yourself the opportunity to get comfortable with the arousal in a controlled way.

Feeling dizzy is a huge problem for anxious people, and it's also a very common sensation that arises when working out. For example, it's quite common to feel a bit dizzy just after stepping off the treadmill. This gives you another sensation to practice with. Your anxious mind might sound the alarm with a *"What if I faint?"* thought, but you reply, "So what! I'll sit down and let it pass. If I do need help, there are plenty of people here to help me." Then you allow the sensation to be there without getting upset by it as you take your rest. Once you're ready, **engage** again with what you're doing. That means really focusing on another exercise and giving it your full attention. By being fully present, you reduce the chances for further anxious thoughts intruding.

What's important is to not overdo any of this. Don't push yourself too fast in the beginning, but rather build your confidence up slowly. After just a few sessions of practicing The DARE Response in this manner, you'll have much greater confidence with any anxious bodily sensation you have in or outside the gym.

THE DARE RESPONSE AT THE DOCTORS/ CHECKING BLOOD PRESSURE

Many people with high anxiety obsess about their blood-pressure reading. Routine tests, such as measuring a patient's blood-pressure level, can cause individuals prone to anxiety to become even more conscious of having an elevated heart rate during the examination (which leads to an unreliable measure of blood pressure). On the whole, doctors are aware of this and have dubbed the condition "white coat syndrome" due to the anxiety-provoking effect the doctors themselves have on some people.

First, it's important to tell your doctor about your anxiety and to explain to them if you're feeling anxious during the examination. Just telling your doctor this can be enough to help you feel more relaxed. If you do discuss your anxiety, be sure to let him or her know about The DARE Response and how you're implementing it. It has been my experience that good doctors are always interested in hearing about non-pharmaceutical approaches that are getting results for their patients.

If your doctor needs to get an accurate blood-pressure measure from you and has been made aware of your anxiety during visits, he or she should suggest an ambulatory blood-pressure-monitoring device (ABPM) that you take with you and that takes blood-pressure readings at regular intervals during the day and night. This device is important because even if you do use The DARE Response in the doctor's office (which I recommend you do anyway), you may still have an aroused nervous system and that can impact test results.

THE DARE RESPONSE FOR TOILET PHOBIA

There are a number of different phobias related to the toilet, but here I'm going to discuss one of the most common: the fear of not getting to the toilet on time. No one should feel ashamed of this problem; it's common and can be overcome. This fear is almost always connected to social embarrassment, and it rarely happens in situations where other people are not around.

Anxiety can give people the impression that they have a weak bladder. When anxious, they may need to use the toilet several times. In most cases, there's no physical problem, and the frequency of needing a toilet is purely psychological.

As with all situational anxiety, "what if" thoughts are the main driver of the fear.

"What if I can't make it to a toilet?" People often run these scenarios through their minds of not being able to reach a toilet on time and the social embarrassment this would cause. If you experience this fear when you leave home, I'll outline steps you can take to minimize the anxiety.

The solution lies in rebuilding confidence in your own body and putting less focus on the fear of embarrassment or ridicule. Start by putting yourself in situations where you know there are toilets, but position yourself far enough away so that your anxiety is activated.

Let's take a shopping mall as an example. As you enter the mall and the fear escalates, find a place to sit down. As the fearful "what if" thoughts surface, defuse them. Simply say to the thoughts, "Whatever. I'm not worried by that scenario because I have full confidence in controlling my body."

You work through The DARE Response by allowing the anxiety to be present. Only when the anxiety lessens, stand up, and then walk slowly and calmly to the toilet. By the time you reach it, you might even find that you no longer need to go.

The important point is to move toward the toilet only when you feel that *you*—not the anxiety—are the one deciding when to go. If you keep running to the toilet every time you feel the urge, you reinforce the idea that you have no control over the situation. By working through the anxiety and going only when you're ready, your confidence in your ability to control your body increases tenfold.

You might want to begin by setting up these opportunities when you're alone. When you're with friends, fear of embarrassment can make it more difficult. As you practice this, you'll reach a point where you feel more confident about controlling your body's need to use the toilet.

THE DARE RESPONSE FOR EATING OUT

We all love to have a nice dinner made by someone else, be it in a restaurant or over at a friend's house, right? Unfortunately, when anxiety creeps in, this is often one of the pleasures it steals from people because several anxious "what ifs" come with a meal.

I want you to now think in your own mind of the "what ifs" and how you might **defuse** those "what ifs."

For example:

"What if I have to leave the restaurant? What will my friends/colleagues think?"

Whatever. I can make up a perfectly normal excuse to leave without a fuss.

"What if I have to leave after my host has gone to so much trouble to prepare a meal? It's so rude!"

So what! It's not the end of the world. If I had to leave, I'd call them the next day to apologize and maybe even send a gift as an apology. They will understand.

"What if my throat feels tight and I feel I can't swallow the food?"

So what? I'll just slowly chew the food and eat what I can. (See the Give up Fearing Sensations chapter for more on this.)

The important thing is to give a firm response and not let these fears stop you from going out for a meal. Always keep pushing out of your comfort zone so that if your partner or friend suggests going out for a meal, just say YES.

As you enter a restaurant, for example, tell yourself you feel excited. "I'm excited by this feeling. I'm excited to be eating out. This is gonna be fun."

As you sit down at the table, **allow** any anxiety you feel to be present. Let it come in waves. Allow it all—the jitters, the restlessness, even the queasy stomach you secretly wished would not manifest but it did. Repeat to yourself, "I accept and allow this anxious feeling. I accept and allow these anxious thoughts."

If your mind keeps coming back to the idea that there is a real threat present, then **run toward** it and tell yourself that you feel really excited to be eating out in a restaurant. Treat it like an adventure.

Try your best to keep focused and **engaged** on the experience. Read the menu, engage in conversation—all the while allowing the anxiety to be.

When you think, "I'm too distracted. I can't enjoy this," take the pressure off yourself to have a good time, and never get upset with yourself. It's okay to not enjoy it. You're recovering from anxiety, and each new situation is a learning experience. The important thing is to do it because the next time you might actually enjoy it like you used to in the past.

One final tip on eating out: Try not to drink too much alcohol. If you really want to drink, have a glass of wine or a beer, but don't overdo it or you'll feel more anxious the next day and might associate that with eating out.

CONCLUSION

What you're learning here is to remove the resistance and fear from situations that have caused you problems in the past. So an overcrowded train becomes exactly that—just an overcrowded train with uncomfortable, heightened bodily sensations. The same for a flight or any other situation that makes you feel tense and on edge. When you remove the fear of fear, your confidence comes bouncing back. Here are some final points and reminders for overcoming anxiety in anxious situations.

GET FAMILIAR WITH THE DARE RESPONSE

Really familiarize yourself with The DARE Response and think in advance how you might apply it in anxious situations that scare you. For example, the night before you're about to take a bus journey, you can rehearse in your mind's eye how you'll handle the waves of anxiety when they manifest. See yourself successfully dealing with the anxiety using each of the steps of The DARE Response. Remember, it's not about doing it without fear; it's doing it with fear and succeeding. This kind of mental rehearsal trains you to respond with greater ease when the situation does occur. You can carry bullet-point notes of The DARE Response with you on a card or on your smartphone when you're out and about so that you can remind yourself how to respond correctly.

MAKE BABY STEPS

Get a journal and create a step-by-step strategy of how you're going to approach the situation you fear. Break it down into small steps that you can manage. Don't try to do too much too soon. If you simply can't motivate yourself to tackle a situation, tell yourself you'll do just a tiny basic step to begin with. For example, with driving, you might start by just driving once around the block then come home. It may be that once you're out and driving, you'll go farther and farther, but the important thing is to make the first step. If elevators are the problem, start by just stepping in one and letting the door close, then get out again. If shopping is the issue, go and buy just one item.

What's important is that you challenge yourself enough so that you do feel some level of anxiety as you put yourself in that situation. If there isn't some level of anxiety, you're probably not pushing out of your comfort zone enough.

IF YOU NEED A SUPPORT PERSON, FIND ONE

Some people can't face the idea of tackling an anxious situation alone. In this case it's fine to bring a support person along with you as you practice The DARE Response and build your confidence up again. Then when you feel ready, you should try doing it alone so that you don't become too dependent on the support person. That person might be your partner or a friend, or it can be a hired person like a therapist who is familiar with this approach of facing anxiety. I know of people who have had driving anxiety that hired a driving instructor to come with them just to get them back out on roads that make them anxious. In this way they felt more comfortable pushing themselves outside their comfort zone.

ALWAYS LEAVE ON YOUR OWN TERMS

Once you've successfully applied The DARE Response to a situation described in this chapter and start to feel more comfortable in that situation, don't immediately turn around and run home. Leaving the situation too soon sends a message that the anxiety might have gotten the better of you if you hadn't left quickly. So as you get more confident, try to stay in the situation until you feel your anxiety decrease. If you can't wait for it to decrease, then at least stay another ten seconds. Just ten seconds more … then maybe another ten seconds after that. Try to win as much ground as you can each time you practice so that you are always building your confidence—even in small incremental steps.

Habituation (getting used to the situation with reduced anxiety) normally takes at least forty-five minutes. So whether you're driving around the block, working out in the gym, or going to the doctor's office, try your best to stay for that period of time. This will really let your anxious mind get the message that this situation is not dangerous. Then when you leave on your own terms—and not anxiety's terms—you'll find your success has really been solidified.

FIND A SIMILAR SITUATION TO PRACTICE WITH

If your real fear is a situation that's not easily practiced, such as flying, find a situation that's somewhat similar. To give you an example, if you fear the claustrophobic feeling you get while flying, then you might start by practicing on an elevator ride where the same fear is triggered. That way you get to build your confidence up slowly and in stages so that when you do get to face your most feared situation, you already have this new skillset practiced and in place.

PUSH THROUGH THE SETBACKS

There will be times it won't work or go as you planned. That's okay too. Those occasions are not failures; they're just the normal part of the recovery process. You can't expect to get it right 100 percent of the time. What's important is that you don't stop trying. As Winston Churchill said, "Never give in, never give in, never; never; never; never."

I hope you've gotten a good understanding of how to apply The DARE Response in different situations. Remember, your anxiety is not in the *situation* itself but rather the *sensations* that you feel. Once you learn to feel more confident with these sensations, the situations will no longer trouble you. I can't emphasize enough how important it is that you go out now and practice! It's only through practice that you'll learn this response to anxiety. For additional support, download the free audios that come with this book.

 visit www.DareResponse.com/app

GIVE UP FEARING ANXIOUS THOUGHTS

We can't control the world around us, we can only control our response to it.

"Stress" is the buzzword of our modern lives. All the media ever seems to talk about is stress. This stress is something done to us. We're given the message that we're all victims of stress because of the fast-paced world we now live in.

No one ever talks about *worry* anymore. It's a word in the therapeutic world that's almost going out of fashion, and I think that's a shame. I much prefer the word "worry" because it reflects a more accurate picture of what's really going on inside our minds and hearts.

General anxiety is not caused by stress—it's caused by worry. We're stressed because we're worried. We're not stressed because we have to drop the kids off, go to work, and earn a living to avoid having the house repossessed. We're stressed because of the way we worry about all of those things. If we didn't worry about any of it, we wouldn't be stressed.

When we can start to talk about worry again, it will clarify the situation better. It places the responsibility of what's happening to us back in our hands. There's less room to blame the world for doing this to us and more room for us to look at our own response to the world.

Every single bit of advice in this book is based on the premise that you, the reader, are responsible for your own destiny and that you can personally take action in your own life to end your anxiety. That's why I prefer to talk about worry because worry is something you can become aware of and then act to change.

Worry is the driving force of general anxiety. The origin of the word worry is actually 'to strangle'. We strangle and contract our lives when we worry. We worry because we think doing so will solve our problems and allow us to feel more in control but it cuts us off from life.

In this chapter I want to talk about the two types of worry that affect people. The **worry over things** and the **worry over thoughts.**

The worry over things is obvious. We worry about our health, the health of our loved ones, money, relationships, careers. We even worry whether we turned the oven off after leaving the house.

The second type of worry is the one that only people with anxiety really suffer from. It's the worry over thoughts. Those are worries about how we think and the thoughts we have. The *"Why can't I stop thinking about such bizarre things?"* type of worry. The second type of worry can turn in on top of itself and prompt a vicious cycle of fearing our thoughts. You can use The DARE Response to handle both types of worries.

Let's look at these two types of worry in more detail.

WORRY OVER THINGS

"Our main business is not to see what lies dimly at a distance, but to do what lies clearly at hand." ~ Thomas Carlyle

I doubt there's anyone alive who doesn't know what it's like to worry. In the West we have turned worry into an art form. We worry about the minor stuff like "*Will I get to the appointment on time?*" to the serious things like "*How will I survive now that I'm out of work?*"

Everyone has different types of worry, and it's all relative to the person that's going through it. What can seem like a disaster to one person can seem like a trivial matter to another. At the deepest level, the one worry almost every human suffers from is a worry about belonging. "*Will I be accepted by my peers/family/society? Will I be loved?*"

Before I discuss how to tackle worry, you first need to ask yourself honestly if you're really willing to give it up. Maybe you actually want to keep worrying because you feel you need it?

Many people are reluctant to let go of worry for fear they'll succumb to some danger. Worry can become a habit that we feel is the only thing keeping us safe and out of harm's way. We rush around in a state of panic from one thing to the next in the false belief that if we slowed down for just a minute, everything would fall apart and it would all be our fault because we dared to stop worrying.

That might seem a bit exaggerated, but nonetheless it's the reality for many people. It's the way our anxious minds work.

Maybe you think that worrying over your career or your finances keeps you more secure? Maybe you think that fear of illness keeps you from doing things that might cause that illness? The reality is that if you actually stopped worrying, you wouldn't be any more or less in danger than you already are.

You would not suddenly miss deadlines or forget to pick up the kids or pay your bills. It's a myth that you need to be driven by worry and fear to get things done. Without worry you'll always have the ability to engage the aspect of your brain that's capable of anticipating future events and problem solving. You don't need to be motivated by worry to become a better person.

Here's how you apply The DARE Response to worry over things:

Let's say for example you have a fear that a loved one might get ill. Maybe they were ill in the past and now you fear that illness might return.

Begin by **defusing** the "what if" worry each time it manifests itself.

"What if his illness comes back? How will we cope then?"

"Oh well, if that happens it happens, we'll have to deal with it, but right now that hasn't happened, so I'm not going to obsess over that right now."

Then **allow** this worry to be present without getting upset by it. Tell yourself that it's perfectly normal to be worried about such things, and don't beat yourself up every time a "what if" thought intrudes.

The "what ifs" may continue to loop, so you'll need to defuse them all the while accepting that such anxiety is normal to feel. If they really loop incessantly, **run toward** them by taking a piece of paper and writing them out over and over. This has a powerful releasing effect.

When that is done, **engage** with something and move your attention fully into what you're doing. If you weren't doing anything in particular before the worry over things arose, find something that engages your attention so that the anxious part of your mind stops obsessing over your fears.

Dale Carnegie wrote a great book on how to deal with this first aspect of worry—the "worry over things"—called *How to Stop Worrying and Start Living*. In it he talks about "shutting the iron doors on the past and the future. Live in Day-tight compartments."

What he means is that we must learn to live in each day and not spend so much time focusing on the past or the future. Regret, for example, is often about things we did or didn't do in the past, and worry is usually about an event in the future.

Carnegie also talks about the fundamental importance of acceptance (the second step of The DARE Response). You have to *"be willing to have it so,"* to accept things as they are, not as you wish they were in this moment. Through acceptance of the challenges you face in life, you melt the tension that worry creates.

If we're presented with a difficult problem, we can wish for the future to be different and make plans to change our situation, but we must first accept reality as it is here and now. So that means if you have lost your job or have just had a health scare, once you have overcome the initial shock of that painful experience, you then need to move into a state of acceptance of it in order to move forward.

Acceptance gives you that starting point from which you can move forward without adding additional worry to the problem. It allows you to start enjoying life while still encountering the challenge that's present. But the challenge now becomes easier because you're actually giving up the most tiring part of any particular challenge, which is the constant worry over it.

The above discussion applies to things that we have no control over; sometimes there are things that we can act upon, and in that case taking action can do a tremendous amount to alleviate the worry.

If there is an action you can take to address your worry, you'll feel more in control and less anxious. So for example, if you've just lost your job, you might go about taking action by doing the following:

1. Write down precisely what you're worried about.

2. Write down what you can do about it.

3. Decide what to do.

4. Start immediately to carry out that decision.

If I ever catch myself worrying over a matter, I determine if this worry is something I can take some decisive action on or if it's a worry about something that's out of my control.

If it's something I can act on, I list the problem and make a note in my smartphone of what needs to happen to resolve this worry. I then write just one step I can take today to move me closer to resolving the issue. I set a reminder to come back to that step later in the day when I have more time to address it properly. Just making these notes helps alleviate the worry.

If it's something that's completely out of my control, I do The DARE Response as outlined above. I defuse the anxious "what if" thoughts through a "whatever" mentality, I accept that this is something I have no control over, and I gently move my attention back to engaging with what I was doing. I may have to do this several times, but inevitably the worry will lose its charge and become less intrusive.

WORRY OVER THOUGHTS

After an extended period of high anxiety, you might find yourself moving from worries over things to worry over thoughts. This is where the creative mind can turn on itself.

The kind of thoughts I'm referring to here are intrusive or disturbing thoughts about subject matters that shock you over just the very fact that you had that particular thought.

Typical intrusive thoughts often revolve around sex or confusion over sexual orientation, blasphemous thoughts, or acting out spontaneously in a violent manner toward loved ones.

People who suffer from frequent intrusive thoughts say things like:

"I can't control them and they really scare me. They keep popping up at random moments."

"What if a part of me wants to do this terrible thing I keep thinking about?"

"What if it's a sign I'm losing control? I feel I have to suppress these thoughts or else they might take over."

It's perfectly normal to start fearing for your sanity or to get upset when intrusive thoughts manifest, but you have to understand they're nothing more than the result of the *elevated stress hormones + mental exhaustion*. The very fact that you're responding with anxiety to these thoughts proves that you're perfectly normal. You're not losing it, nor are you a bad person for thinking them. You're just suffering from the side effects of high anxiety.

Thinking happens ... and it's not who you are.

A thought is just a thought—it's not a fact. The fact that you think something doesn't make it so, nor does it reflect on the person you are. *Don't mistake the content of your thoughts for the person you are.* These thoughts don't represent the real you.

On average we have about 50,000 thoughts every day. Many of these are bizarre and wacky. We all have them. The only difference is that when you're feeling highly sensitized, those thoughts really stand out and grab your attention. You then feel a jolt of fear like an electrical *zap* when you respond to them in horror.

For example, driving the kids to school you might have an out-of-the-blue thought: *"What if I just swerved into this on coming car?"*

Zap! You react in terror and feel the jolt of fear in your stomach.

That thought alone is enough to knock the wind right out of you. *"How could I ever think such a thing?* I must be going mad!"

Zap, zap!

All of this self-doubt and fear leads to more anxious thoughts, and you're back in that vicious cycle of anxiety.

Other typical examples might be:

"What if I just jumped off this balcony ...?"

"What if I actually don't love my partner anymore ...?"

"What if I did something totally inappropriate right now ...?"

Everyone's initial response is to react in fear to such thoughts and then try to push them away, but this is the key mistake we all make.

The harder you push those thoughts away from your mind, the harder they bounce back.

Remember as a child when you played with an inflatable beach ball in the pool? Every time you tried to push it down under the water to sit on it, it just kept springing back up with the same force you used to keep it down, often hitting you on the face.

The same goes for these intrusive thoughts. You simply can't expect to get peace from them by pushing them away. The only way to get peace is to allow that beach ball to float along beside you. You must stop responding with fear to the thoughts that terrify you and learn to accept and allow them.

When I say "accept and allow" an intrusive thought, I don't mean that you agree with the content of the thought. I mean that you accept the thought for what it is, a random thought generated by an anxious mind and nothing more.

Let me give you an example of how you can apply The DARE Response to these intrusive thoughts. Remember, you can't control intrusive thoughts or worries; you can control only your response to them.

Let's say for example that you're cutting the vegetables for dinner, and your partner walks into the kitchen and gets something out of the fridge.

As they have their back to you, an intrusive thought crosses your mind: *"What if I lost control and stabbed him/her in the back with this knife?"*

The old you would have felt a jolt of terror punch you in the stomach and maybe even scare you enough to have to put the knife back in the drawer. The new you, using the philosophy of The DARE Response, doesn't put the knife down but keeps chopping and begins by **defusing** the anxious "what if."

"What if I just randomly stabbed him/her with this knife?"

"Oh well, *then I'd get locked up. At least I wouldn't have to make dinner anymore!*"

You defuse the anxious thought by being flippant or humorous toward it, instead of being scared by it. Use whatever response you feel achieves that goal. It's a bit like the way you might respond to a small child who comes into the room dressed as a monster trying to scare you. "Oh, you're so big and scary!" you say with wry smile.

Then **allow** the intrusive thought to be present without any resistance. Let it stay for as long as it likes. Remember the beach ball example. If you try to push it down, it will bounce back, so let it be present and then gently move your attention back to what you were doing. On occasion, when you're feeling quite anxious, some thoughts can have a highly persistent nature. I call it a "high glue factor" as they really stick to you! This is where you can implement the "run toward" step of The DARE Response. Instead of just acknowledging and accepting the thought, you can get excited and demand more of it to really shake yourself loose of its grip.

"Oh that's a weird idea again of doing something totally inappropriate. It seems very strong today. Okay—so let's have it! I'm going to think about this all day. Come on, let's see if I can think of even stranger things than that."

Lastly, e**ngage** with whatever is at hand. In this case, you move your attention back to making the dinner all the while not pushing the thought away.

With very intrusive thoughts you may have to do the above steps several times in a row each time the intrusive thoughts grab a hold of you. Once you remove the emotional response to intrusive thoughts, you normalize them and they no longer have an emotional pull. When they no longer have a pull, they fall away by themselves naturally as they have nothing to cling onto.

YOU ARE NOT THOSE THOUGHTS

These intrusive thoughts don't represent the real you. They're just the result of your creative imagination mixed with anxiety and exhaustion. In fact, rather than beat yourself up over them, you can congratulate yourself on your creative ability!

These thoughts love a good, fearful response to keep them going. They're a bit like an annoying bee buzzing about; it's usually only when we try to swat at it that it stings us back. When you let them be, they buzz off in their own time. The mental tension you feel will dissipate very fast if you can adopt this attitude of nonresistance to these intrusive thoughts.

I'm not suggesting this is something easy to do. It takes practice to retrain yourself not to respond with fear to such thoughts. As you progress, you'll no longer respond in fear to certain thoughts, but new, strange ones might catch you off guard. If that happens, you need to keep applying and practicing The DARE Response each and every time they arrive and never beat yourself up if you don't always do it perfectly.

There will be times it will be easy to do, and then there will be moments when you're tired and feeling vulnerable and the thoughts just get the upper hand. That's just how it is sometimes.

Practice and practice and eventually you'll get it.

CONCLUSION

In closing this chapter, here are two helpful ways to visualize anxious thoughts. They're popular visual cues used in cognitive behavioral therapy and tie in well with the steps of The DARE Response.

CLOUDS PASSING OVERHEAD

Imagine yourself lying on your back in a field watching the clouds pass overhead. Some of these clouds are white and puffy while others are dark and ominous. Each cloud represents a thought. You're the passive observer just watching as each one of them floats by—and they always float by.

Watching your thoughts in a detached manner allows you to not judge any of the clouds or get sucked in. You're the silent observer, just watching. Label each thought as you become aware of it (**defuse it**), "Oh, there's that weird thought X again—oh well," and then just let it float on past (**allow it**). As they float away, tell some of the more troubling or disturbing thoughts to come back (**run toward**). When you get bored doing this, place your attention back on an activity that holds your attention (**engage**).

SOCK PUPPETS

Picture your anxious "what if" thoughts, your worries over thoughts, like sock puppets that are up close and in your ear telling you all manner of scary or worrying things. If you really visualize the ridiculous nature of these sock puppets, it lessens the emotional impact of the thoughts so that you can more easily dismiss the content of the thoughts as being irrelevant or nonsense (thereby **defusing** them). Treat these sock puppets with tolerance, even compassion (**allow**), but don't take them seriously for one second. The more dismissive you can be about the things these sock puppets tell you, the easier it is for you to drop the fearful resistance of them. If you really want to strip them of any fear, chase after them (**run toward**). Tell them to stay around for as long as possible. When you're bored with the exercise, focus on something else that **engages** you.

Important Side Note:

I find intrusive thoughts act like a barometer of your anxiety levels. They manifest at the lower ends of the anxiety scale. They're often the first thing to show up before bodily sensations and are also the last thing you'll notice when you're close to a full recovery. When people tell me that they have everything else under control except for their intrusive, anxious thoughts, I know this is a sign they're making good progress and are very close to a full recovery.

GIVE UP YOUR SAFE ZONE

The day came when the risk to remain tight in a bud was more painful than the risk it took to blossom.

-Anaïs Nin

Now that we're farther into the book, I want you to push yourself even further and really challenge yourself to bravely step outside your safe zone. That's where the real learning and progress happens.

Every anxious person has a safe zone they feel comfortable in. That safe zone may be familiar environments like their home or their neighborhood, or they can be anywhere that they're with a support person who understands and helps them. Safe zones appear to help us feel reassured that everything's manageable. The problem is that they're a self-imposed prison.

Because comfort is found there, it's where the person tends to spend more and more time. The problem with anxiety is that it tends to encroach on everything until eventually the safe zone becomes just the four walls of a person's home (agoraphobia).

The safe zone is a myth. In reality there's no such thing as a safe zone from anxiety. As there's nothing life-threatening about a panic attack, you're not in any more danger sitting at home than you are sitting out under the stars in the outback of Australia. Of course, your mind immediately rushes to tell you that the outback of Australia is a ridiculous place to be because there are no hospitals, no tranquilizers, no doctors, NO SAFETY.

Review your previous experiences of anxiety and panic attacks. Aren't you still here, alive and well, after all those attacks during which you were convinced you were going to die?

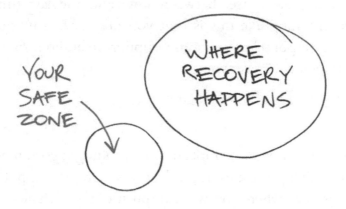

You may have been driven, on occasion, to the hospital, where they did medicate you to calm you down. But do you really believe that you wouldn't have survived were it not for the drugs? You would have. If the same bout of anxiety had occurred in the middle of nowhere and you were all alone, it would have passed as well. Yes, when it comes to conditions that need medical attention—such as asthma, diabetes, and a whole litany of other conditions—then having medical aid nearby is a big asset. But no doctor in the world would tell someone with anxiety that there are only specific safe zones in which he or she can move.

So I want you to now really push outside your safe zone. Cross that red line in your mind and go for it. I want you to dig really deep and push out like you've never done before. *It's never enough to just read what you need to do; you have to experience it.* Real growth and learning happen when we challenge ourselves, when we feel the anxiety and push beyond our comfort levels. As Susan Jeffers wrote, we have to "feel the fear and do it anyway."

Are you willing to feel the fear today?

I know more than anyone how terrifying it can feel to move out of your safe zone as the fear wells up inside, but you have what it takes to do this. I know you're strong enough. You wouldn't have read this far into the book if you weren't.

The difference, of course, between now and the last time you attempted anything like this is that you now have a unique tool (The DARE Response) as well as my support in audio form for you to take with you wherever you go.

visit www.DareResponse.com/app

I'm going to give you an example of how you might go about doing this. I'll use driving as the example, but this example is applicable to any circumstance where you want to push out and challenge your safe zone.

As I mentioned previously with driving, it's important to break this challenge up into steps so that you keep pushing yourself a bit farther each day. That might mean driving to the end of your street on your first attempt and then around the block the next day.

As you drive and feel the anxiety, you implement The DARE Response, and then once you notice that you're a significant way outside your safe zone, pull over and stay there. Work through the anxiety in that new space.

Don't just turn around and rush home. Rushing home sends the signal that you *just* made it, but if you stayed any longer, you might have gotten yourself into some trouble. That's not true, and you need to counteract those fears by proving to yourself that you can really stay outside your safe zone just fine. Sure, it might be uncomfortable, but hold your ground and don't retreat.

Leave on your own terms—not anxiety's. Stay in the new location until you no longer feel anxious. That way you firmly plant your flag of success in the ground and claim that new territory as yours. You're outside your old safe zone, and even though you felt anxious, you stayed there and worked through it. Now you can return home with a much greater sense of confidence regarding what you accomplished. You left your safe zone and achieved your objective. That's a real success.

Once you get home, solidify the success by writing it down in your journal. This is very important to make it all the more real. Then immediately write down what your next goal is going to be.

Maybe you're going to drive a few blocks farther? Maybe you're going to try driving in traffic? You can do it the following day if you feel ready for it or give yourself one day's break. The important thing is to not leave it more than a few days, or anxiety will creep in and steal that ground back from you. Don't let it. Keep going and always be pushing this invisible boundary out farther.

If you keep this momentum going, the illusion of a safe zone will suddenly evaporate. You'll start to feel really safe and secure within yourself no matter where you are, be it out in the wilderness or in a crowded place or even flying over the Atlantic. That freedom comes from pushing through any setback and never giving up. It varies from person to person exactly when that happens, but you can be guaranteed that if you stick at it, you'll get there.

Yes, you're allowed to have days off, of course. I don't want you to push yourself too hard if you feel you're not ready for it. There will be days when you just don't feel up to it and want to hide under the covers. That's okay; allow for those down days, but then once your energy returns, pick yourself up and get out there again. Build up the psychological momentum again and be relentless.

Keep pushing through!

I know some of you might be thinking that you can't practice your particular fear easily because it's hard to replicate (e.g., flying or public speaking), but there are ways to put yourself in situations that trigger a similar fear in which you can practice. For example, a man I coached who had a claustrophobic fear of sitting in an airplane would use elevators in tall skyscrapers to practice working through his fear. Another man who wanted to overcome his anxiety of talking at work meetings used a weekly Toastmasters club to practice his delivery. Be creative. There are always ways to come up with situations that you know will trigger a similar anxiety for you in which you can challenge yourself.

If you want a fast recovery, it's found outside your safe zone, experiencing the anxiety and working through it. It's so much better to be out there in the world, feeling anxious and working through it, than living in an imagined bubble of safety.

When you push outside your safe zone, *don't expect to enjoy it*, even if it's a fun thing like going to the cinema or eating out with friends. Treat it like homework. In the early days it will just feel uncomfortable as you'll be so focused on the challenge, but as you continue to practice, you'll eventually start to enjoy doing it.

Take a moment now and make the decision to do this. I want you to really go after this like your life depends on it. Is there anything more important you could be working toward? You're fighting to win back your very freedom.

Take The DARE Response audio with you when you push outside your comfort zone. Have me there with you supporting you through each challenge. Get the free audio now at www.DareResponse.com/audio

GIVE UP BEING SO HARD ON YOURSELF

People who suffer from anxiety tend to be incredibly hard on themselves. The longer the anxiety is present, the worse this gets. These people would not give themselves such a hard time if they suffered from a physical malady like diabetes, but they sure do abuse themselves for having a mental health issue like anxiety.

I think the reason for this is that part of them believes that it's their fault. There's an accompanying shame of feeling weak for being susceptible to fear and anxiety. Once this kind of negative self-talk creeps in, it can lead to feelings of depression and loneliness. Patrick, who has been a great contributor to my coaching program, calls it the "collateral damage" he used to do to himself daily after each episode of anxiety.

I bet that you're a very kind person. The only problem is that you might not be so kind to yourself. You might be your own worst critic. Why is that? Why do we treat others so much better than we treat ourselves? If your best friend was suffering from anxiety, I'm sure you'd be encouraging and supportive and wouldn't dream of saying the kind of things you tell yourself daily.

As another coaching member put it:

"I've had counseling for three years, and it was always pointed out to me how hard I am on myself. The kindness and generosity I've shown to others is never there for myself."

So where does this intense self-criticism come from? Most of it, in my opinion, is fueled by a simple lie. The lie is that you're not good enough. It's that simple. You feel that you're defective in some way and not worthy. When you believe this lie, you fear getting rejected or abandoned by others for not being good enough.

Most of the human race believes this selfsame lie, and as a result many of us suffer from low self-esteem. This is the reason that public speaking is often cited as peoples' number one fear because public speaking opens us up to immediate rejection.

This one single lie—that you aren't good enough—is the cause of so much unhappiness and, in extreme cases, even hatred of oneself. When things go wrong, like when anxiety manifests, that problem of low self-worth becomes magnified.

In this short chapter I'm going to focus on the solution. As you'll have gathered by now, I only recommend simple and effective psychological approaches that can be easily implemented.

Every therapy has its own series of steps and procedures to tackle low self-esteem. The most popular therapy today (CBT) would approach this problem by having the person learn to identify and replace destructive negative thought patterns with more healthy and productive ones.

Although this can be effective, I think this therapeutic approach often fails to address low self-esteem issues because of the continuous effort required to monitor and replace these destructive thoughts. After a week or two, people tend to lose patience with the exercise because of the tiring effort involved. The other reason this approach fails many people is that it doesn't go deep enough into the heart of the problem. It fails to tackle the lie that's buried deep within the person's psyche. It's more like a gardener only snipping what he can see of a weed instead of pulling it up by the roots.

What works much better is finding a really simple technique that has the power to end this lie by rewiring your level of self-worth. This chapter goes beyond the scope of just healing anxiety and touches the area of transformational self-development. If you feel this isn't something you want to look at right now, then feel free to skip it, but please do consider coming back to it at a later stage because of the profound effect this exercise can have on the quality of your life.

Since I was a teenager, I've had a keen interest in personal development. I've attended countless self-development workshops and seminars around the world and read hundreds of books on the subject. Having worked in the self-help space helping people with anxiety for over ten years, I've had the opportunity to meet many great teachers as well as a handful of charlatans. The amount of time I've invested in studying personal growth material hasn't transformed me into an enlightened person by any stretch of the imagination, but it has given me the ability to quickly discern between approaches that work and those that don't.

I'm not exaggerating when I say that what follows may be the most powerful self-help exercise you'll come across. There are many different versions of this same exercise, and many authors have books on it, but the take I like the most comes from Kamal Ravikan's book *Love Yourself*. He keeps the exercise so simple, and as a result it's mightily powerful.

THE EXERCISE

During any free moment you have, repeat this sentence to yourself: "I love myself."

Repeat it when you wake in the morning over and over. Say it while you're brushing your teeth, eating your breakfast, on the way to work.

Fill every idle moment in your day with this one same mantra. "I love myself. I love myself. I love myself."

That's it!

Be careful not to overlook this as too idiotic.

Bear in mind that the biggest fear people have is not to be loved. To be ostracized, rejected, or betrayed is what troubles people deep down the most. We all crave love, but for various reasons we don't get the level of love that we need.

We are in fact hardwired for love. When you repeat the words "I love myself" like a mantra, it's so simple that it slips past the analysis of our conscious mind and travels straight down to that deeper subconscious level within us where we hold our core beliefs about ourselves. There it ever so slowly dismantles the lie we've been telling ourselves and replaces it with a more positive self-image.

The beauty of this practice is that there's no need to consciously create something positive. You don't have to force anything. You don't have to worry about monitoring and correcting each and every negative thought. Skip the years of therapy trying to come to terms with all the love that was withheld from you. Give it to yourself now and in each and every moment you find your mind idle.

In the beginning you probably won't believe that you really love yourself, but that doesn't matter. Just keep doing it until the message seeps so far down that it overrides the lie of your low self-worth.

Turn this exercise into a ritual. A daily practice. You can't do it for just a few days and hope to see a change. You have to incorporate it into your life completely.

Say to yourself:

"From this day on I vow to love myself and to treat myself as someone I truly value. Each decision I make from now on will be based on this perspective."

Stop waiting for the world to love you. We have to respect, appreciate, and love ourselves first and foremost. Choose to love yourself.

So through it all, keep repeating to yourself, *"I love myself."*

Don't try to find a reason to justify your love. Instead, give your love to yourself unconditionally and without reserve. You don't need a reason, and you don't need anyone to say you deserve it. Choose to love yourself unapologetically.

So walking to work, you say, *"I love myself."* Waiting for money to come out of the ATM: *"I love myself."* Cleaning the dishes: *"I love myself."* Driving your car: *"I love myself."* Repeat it over and over. What better thought could you ever have going through your head?

Each time you practice, it's like giving yourself a small but precious gift. Go about your day "love bombing" your subconscious mind. This has the effect of literally rewiring the neurological pathways of how you think and perceive yourself.

You'll soon start to abandon old patterns, thoughts, and beliefs that no longer align with this new self-image you're creating. Eventually your mind will release the core lie, and you'll just start to feel better about yourself without having to make any conscious effort at all. Then you'll notice a change in your life and in the way people behave toward you.

Little things will start to happen that never happened before. People will smile at you spontaneously, and your interaction with the world will change for the better. This happens because you're communicating a message about yourself all the time, and much of what we communicate is nonverbal—the way we look at people, the way we hold our bodies, the tones we use. People pick up on this message. If the message that you're sending is one that says "I value myself," people start to unconsciously respond differently to you.

Love yourself and life will respond in kind.

Philip McKernan writes, "*We give ourselves what we feel we deserve.*"

I think there is truth in that. So much of what goes on in our lives reflects the way we feel about ourselves deep down. If we feel we don't deserve something, we often find a way to unconsciously prevent ourselves from getting it.

How many people have you seen sabotage their own happiness? You look on in disbelief, wondering why on earth they'd behave in such a blatantly self-destructive way. An example of this might be a self-destructive habit or addiction or destroying a perfectly good marriage for a meaningless affair.

Having a low sense of self-worth can also manifest as an inability to stand up for what you believe in, an inability to say no, or just letting great opportunities pass you by—all because deep down the lie inside dictates that you don't deserve to be happy.

But isn't saying "I love myself" an incredibly narcissistic thing to think?

No, it's not. Don't fall for that age-old trap. This isn't about becoming arrogant, conceited, or vain in any way. It's about giving yourself what you need in order to love and serve others better. How can you be there for others if you aren't there for yourself?

Kamal puts it well in his book when he compares it to the preflight safety drill you see before take off. If oxygen masks drop from above during the flight, you have to put yours on first before you help your children with theirs. You're no good to them passed out.

I know many of you reading this might be thinking this exercise is too corny, but I'm convinced that years from now some scientists will discover exactly why a simple technique like this works so well. It may come down to the interaction of certain hormones, or maybe it will have something to do with the neuroplasticity of the brain, or it might be something more transcendental.

Who knows? What I do know is that you have absolutely nothing to lose in trying it. Worst-case scenario? It will just be a waste of your time! But then, what were you thinking to yourself anyway that was so important while you were brushing your teeth or clearing out the garbage?

When you consider that the nature of mind is thought, why not fill your mind with the most transformative and powerful thought available to you?

I dare you from this day forward to love yourself fiercely!

Here is a meditative version of this same practice that you can do before you fall asleep or when you wake up in the morning.

Start by taking some deep belly breaths.

Belly breaths are ones that lift your stomach instead of your chest.

Imagine you're breathing down into your legs. Breathe in until you feel full, hold it for a few seconds, and then breathe out slowly.

As you're breathing in, I want you to imagine that you're inside a waterfall of white light. The bright light is falling from high above. The water is illuminated with a brilliant intensity. Feel it pouring over the top of your head and down your arms and legs.

On each in-breath say to yourself, "I love myself."

Hold for a few seconds, and then, as you breathe out, feel all the tension release. Imagine the waterfall again pouring over you, washing away tension and stress.

So for example:

In-breath: "I love myself."

Hold

Out-breath: Feel the tension flow away.

You're going to feel a strong resistance to this exercise when you first start practicing. Expect that. I want you to use The DARE Response to work through this resistance in the exact same manner as you do with anxiety when it manifests.

The resistance you feel during this exercise might be a physical sensation of unease or a series of negative thoughts, like:

"Love myself? Are you kidding? Don't you remember all your shortcomings?

No? Well, let me list them out for you again."

1. I want you to start by defusing any negative thoughts with a strong "so what" or "whatever" response so that these thoughts don't escalate or suck you in.

(e.g., "Whatever. I know I'm not perfect, but I can love myself nevertheless.")

Or

"So what? I love how imperfect I am. It feels more real to me."

2. Then allow any physical resistance you feel to just be there with you as you continue doing the exercise. Don't force it away. Just try to get comfortable with that discomfort as you continue the exercise.

3. Move your full attention back onto the exercise and keep breathing in and out.

In-breath: "I love myself."

Hold

Out-breath: Feel the tension flow away.

You're going to continue the exercise for a minimum of seven minutes. Anything shorter than that won't get the desired stress-reducing effect. (Of course, please keep going with it for longer if you wish.)

GIVE UP FEARING IT WILL LAST FOREVER

> "Hope is like a bird that senses the dawn and carefully starts to sing while it is still dark."
>
> –Anonymous

When in the mire of anxiety, one of the most predominant fears is that the experience will last forever. This prison without walls will become a permanent reality in your life. You project into the future and can see only misery, having to always live with the restriction and avoidance that fear of anxiety creates.

When you're in the throes of such depressing emotions, you can soften that emotion with this one thought:

This too shall pass.

And it will.

Shervin Pishevar wrote, "Fear is finite, hope is infinite." You have to maintain your faith and hope that your circumstance will change. When you least expect it, things will get better.

You may not believe it right now, but the person you dream of, the one willing to go anywhere you want, to do anything you want, is there waiting under all of those anxious feelings. Those anxious feelings blow through like storms, but this storm you feel will run out of rain. No matter how dark and turbulent, they eventually clear and the bright-blue sky appears again.

It's wonderful to watch how the sky and clouds go dark just before the break of dawn, as if heralding some great event that will take place from out of nowhere. It's often the same with recovery from anxiety. Just when you think it's at its worst, you get the breakthrough that you were looking for. If you can't see clearly just now, hold fast and wait for the breaking of the day.

Don't give up!

People frequently ask me if I experience anxiety anymore. It's a good question because if you've been suffering from constant anxiety or panic attacks, you want to get an idea of what full recovery looks like, or if a full recovery is ever possible.

Life is stressful and anxiety will always be a part of our lives, but the difference is I don't get caught in the anxiety loop, and therefore it doesn't develop into a "disorder" anymore. Let me digress briefly and tell you about a real storm I was recently caught up in that helps explain this point.

My wife is Brazilian, and we've been fortunate to be able to visit and explore her amazing country on several occasions. On one particular trip we were on the Amazon River in a small wooden canoe with some other tourists and a fourteen-year-old boy acting as our guide.

In situations like that, where you're surrounded by fish with sharp teeth and nowhere to disembark, it's normal to have a flash fear come to mind. "What if I really want to get off? What if something happens to the canoe? What if? What if? What if?"

I immediately noticed how I had been baited by the anxiety, so I implemented The DARE Response. Within seconds the flash fear subsided, and I was back to feeling excited and ready. I moved out of a possible anxious state and engaged with the moment. The old me could have easily gotten into a state of high anxiety or panic, but armed with The DARE Response in a situation like that, I had a new empowered response.

As it turns out, something did in fact happen, but because of The DARE Response, I was in the perfect state of mind to respond to it. Our young guide had taken us too far downstream and wasn't paying attention to how late it was. As it turns out, it rains very heavily every day in the afternoon, and it's not a good idea to be in a canoe with that many people when it rains. To make matters worse, none of us were wearing a life jacket.

As we turned the canoe to head home, heavy rain started to fall. This was an unusually heavy downpour; each drop looked the size of a marble! You could barely see your hand in front of your face. Below us swam a school of hungry piranha fish.

There was a scramble to put cameras in protective plastic bags, and my wife turned to our guide and asked if it was safe to be out in this kind of rain. His worried little face said it all. "Não!" (No!)

It took only about one minute before the canoe held an inch or two of water and if it kept filling like that we would soon capsize. The vegetation on each side was too thick to disembark, so getting home fast was the only option. During all of this I never felt anxiety overwhelm me; rather I was able to keep my mind clear in a moment of real emergency.

In the end, it was a large empty bottle of Coke that saved us. Myself and a Japanese student took the initiative to cut the Coke bottle in half with a penknife and then we used both ends to bail the water out as fast as it was coming in. We bailed water that afternoon like Olympic sportsmen. With that team effort, we managed to keep the water from rising above our ankles and eventually made it back to the lodge.

Our guide was clearly shook but relieved when we made it back. He tried to make light of it to his anxious father who was waiting for us on the jetty. The rest of us disembarked, relieved to be alive and in need of a stiff Caipirinha. The reason I am telling you this story is not to brag but to show that when you decide to have a new response to your anxiety, you empower yourself to act better in any situation. It's also nice to play MacGyver sometimes!

SETBACKS AND HOW TO DEAL WITH THEM

When a person starts making some good progress in his or her relationship with anxiety, a new "what if" fear creeps in.

"What if the anxiety returns?"

"What if I get thrown back into my prison cell of anxiety?"

This fear is very common. It's understandable to doubt your newfound freedom. In fact, it's almost guaranteed that you'll have a major setback. *I've mentored very few people to freedom who have <u>not</u> had setbacks during their recovery.* There is an old English proverb that says *"a smooth sea never made a skillful sailor."* Setbacks are like final-stage exams you have to pass through in order to earn your freedom.

Setbacks are particularly common after you've had a significant breakthrough, such as doing something that you were previously anxious about, e.g., overcoming a major obstacle or after a significant life event like moving home, changing jobs, etc.

As it's almost a guarantee that you'll experience setbacks, you should expect them and welcome them! If you fully understand that setbacks are part of the healing process, you can drop the frustration you feel and move through them with greater speed.

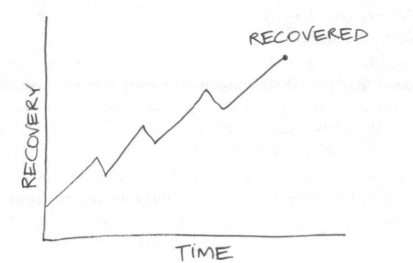

The most upsetting thing about having a setback is the shock it gives you. There you were, making great progress, and then suddenly from out of the blue—the anxiety hits you hard. You not only feel like you're back at square one, but you now fear you'll *never* be free of anxiety and that any advances you made were all an illusion.

Dr. Reid Wilson talks about the importance of learning to "love the mat." It's a martial arts expression that means you have to expect to get thrown to the floor every now and then. When you expect it, you don't get upset by it. Instead, you actually learn to appreciate that it's all part of the experience of growth and learning. It makes you stronger.

Learning to retrain how you respond to setbacks is key. The wrong response prolongs the setback. The right response moves you through it with much greater ease. The right response is The DARE Response.

Start by **defusing** the anxious "what ifs" that arise.

What if all the progress I made was an illusion? What if I never get rid of this? What if I've made my anxiety worse by trying to end it?

Defuse each of these questions with a strong dismissive statement, such as:

"Well, whatever. Then I guess I'll just feel anxious if that's the way it's going to be today."

Next, **allow** the setback to be; don't fight it. In fact, welcome it and see it as part of your continued growth. Let go of wanting uncomfortable anxiety gone and accept and allow it to be exactly as it is today. Allow yourself to have this setback. Remember, it's not forever. Everything changes, and this storm will pass.

Finally, when you're ready, stop focusing on the setback and **engage** with something to keep your anxious mind from ruminating on the setback.

WORK WITH YOUR PROTECTIVE SELF

Setbacks often happen because, as you face your anxiety, the protective side of your personality that would rather you left well enough alone becomes active. Your protective side is the one that wants to stay in its comfort zone with the illusion that you're safe there. Why even put yourself in a situation that makes you feel anxious?

We all know deep down that a life free from adversity isn't possible—and it certainly doesn't lead to happiness. Yet your protective side fears that signs of adversity mean a great fall must be just around the corner. Your protective side doesn't want to defuse, allow, or engage. "Whoa! Whoa!" says your protective self. "What are you doing? Are you crazy? You can't be pushing outside your safe zone like that!" Instead, it wants to put on the brakes and retreat!

Well, we know what happens then: this resistance actually creates a conflict and fuels feelings of anxiety. Your feelings now can be very intense and might be similar to what you've experienced before—such as panic and general unease—or there may be new sensations never experienced before. You might have been doing really well for a while, but then your protective side pops its head up and says something like this:

"No panic attacks for a week—great. But you know what that means ... a really BIG one is waiting in store for you!"

These thoughts undermine your confidence. You feel vulnerable again as the setback tries to convince you that you're not making progress. Anxiety returns, your confidence dips, and you return to obsessing about the way you feel.

You always have to remember that setbacks are part of your healing. They may feel like a big step backward, but they're followed by rapid progress on many levels.

To move beyond the anxiety, you need to create a new working relationship with your protective self—this will really seal your recovery. Educate your protective self that you're really safe and encourage it to take these steps with you so that you become fully empowered to end your anxiety problem. When you do, all your internal energies go in the same direction, and there's no longer any conflict.

The other important thing to do is to release the frustration you feel. The frustration of feeling stuck again. The frustration of not been 100 percent better yet. Don't hate your setbacks—embrace them as opportunities for further growth.

Drop the frustration you feel by really accepting that what you're experiencing right now is a necessary part of the healing process. Don't beat yourself up over it, and appreciate that the journey you're on is special to you alone. You need to be kind to yourself. Understand that these setbacks are the result of you just trying to protect you. Be your own best friend.

Recovery is not a linear process like healing a broken bone. Some days will be better than others—that's just the way it is, so don't get upset if you complete something successfully one day but fail the next. Keep your eyes on the end goal, and persistence will carry you there.

Whenever you find yourself doubting your recovery, remember how far you've come. Remember all the anxiety you've faced, all the fears you've overcome.

Build your confidence by keeping a success diary that describes all the times you successfully dealt with your anxiety. This diary can become an invaluable resource from which to draw strength. Writing down successes not only helps you remember them, but it solidifies them and makes them more real in your mind. We all tend to forget our achievements, so having a record of them is a powerful tool to have at your disposal anytime you need a boost of reassurance and confidence. Confidence, just like fear, is contagious. Soon you'll find it spreading to all areas of your life, giving you a quality of life even beyond your pre-anxiety days.

Yes, sometimes setbacks will hit so hard that you'll feel like you're losing against anxiety. That's okay. Everyone has those days where you just want to hit the snooze button and stay under the covers. Those low points are to be expected. Prepare for them and promise yourself that you'll keep moving forward whenever they occur.

The last word on that has to go to none other than Rocky Balboa:

"You, me, or nobody is gonna hit as hard as life. But it ain't about how hard you hit. It's about how hard you can get hit and keep moving forward; how much you can take and keep moving forward. That's how winning is done!"

GIVE UP SEEING THIS AS A CURSE

"The wound is the place where the Light enters you."

– Rumi

In Japan there's an ancient technique of repairing objects called *Kintsugi*. It's the art of repairing broken ceramic bowls instead of discarding them. They fill the cracks with a gold-speckled resin so that when the bowl is repaired, it makes it more beautiful and valuable than before.

Your anxiety is the crack through which you become a more beautiful person.

Elisabeth Kübler-Ross wrote: "The most beautiful people we have known are those who have known defeat, known suffering, known struggle, known loss, and have found their way out of the depths. These persons have an appreciation, a sensitivity, and an understanding of life that fills them with compassion, gentleness, and a deep loving concern. Beautiful people do not just happen."

I'm going to explain why anxiety, when embraced, can actually be something that can transform you for the better, how it can have a very positive meaning and purpose in your life. In order to get to that stage, you need to have a new perception of it. That new perception comes from applying *forgiveness, meaning, and gratitude.*

1. Forgiveness

2. Meaning

3. Gratitude

1. FORGIVENESS

Most people hate their anxiety and maybe you do, too. You didn't ask for this burden to be heaped upon you, and yet here it is in your life causing total havoc. You have all kinds of other things that you have to manage, and anxiety is the last thing you need to worry about right now.

You might wake some mornings and wonder:

"Why me?"

"What did I do to deserve this?"

"I wish it would just **** off and leave me in peace."

Right?

Anxiety can be such a demoralizing experience, and as we have seen, it often leads to feelings of depression as you think about facing each day with the challenges it brings. I understand how frustrating that can feel as I've felt it too. It's also very normal to feel angry with yourself as we discussed in the last chapter. If this resonates with you, if you notice a strong resentment toward the anxiety, then it's important to be aware of that in order to move forward.

The first step is to become aware of it. Awareness is the first step to solving any problem.

Now, with this awareness, I'm going to ask you to consider forgiving yourself for anxiety and even forgiving the anxiety itself for intruding in your life. The acceptance you've been learning about in The

DARE Response has forgiveness at its core. If you really come to accept a thing, you learn to forgive it for any trouble it causes you.

Forgiving your anxiety means forgiving its unwanted intrusions at exactly the wrong moment. Forgiving the way it startles you in the middle of the night. Forgiving it for never giving you a moment's peace. I know how hard it is to forgive something that's tormented you so much, but it's through forgiveness that you empower yourself and rise above it.

The way to start the forgiveness process is to begin by simply noticing any resentment you hold toward your anxiety and possibly toward yourself. Then just sit with that feeling for a while. Acknowledge and label it for what it is. You're not going to try to do anything with it; just allow it to be present. This way you become mindful of it.

Then ask yourself if you would be willing to forgive yourself and the anxiety?

If you feel you hold most of the anger toward yourself, then look at yourself in a mirror and tell yourself:

"I forgive you for having anxiety."

Speak the words out loud.

Try to feel the same way you would toward a dear friend who was going through the same experience. Talk to yourself in that same manner. What would you say to them? How would you get them to stop beating themselves up over it?

Forgiveness is not a switch you flick and then it's suddenly there. It's something you nurture and cultivate over time. To stay motivated you should remind yourself from time to time why you're nurturing forgiveness. Here are three compelling reasons for you to consider i:

-**Forgiveness is a gift you give yourself.** Louis Smedes once said, "To forgive is to set a prisoner free and discover that the prisoner was you."

Holding resentment toward anxiety limits your ability to truly accept the anxiety and therefore limits the healing effect of The DARE Response. You'll heal your anxiety much faster if you allow yourself to receive the gift of forgiveness because forgiveness is a gift you give to yourself, first and foremost. Any moment—no matter how brief—that you move into forgiveness, you're healing your anxiety.

-**Forgiveness is the real you.** Forgiveness is an act of strength, and it comes from the more grounded version of yourself, that strong person that you're the most proud of.

Mahatma Gandhi said, "*The weak can never forgive. Forgiveness is the attribute of the strong.*"

As you move into forgiveness, you reinforce the wiser, stronger part of you and get to live more fully with a greater sense of wholeheartedness and flow.

-**Forgiveness brings you peace of mind.** Peace of mind comes from letting go of anger and resentment. When you say to yourself, "It's time to forgive this anxiety. It's time to forgive myself for my perceived failings," that's when peace drops in.

Resentment and anger toward yourself or your anxiety don't serve you. They rob you of your energy and keep you feeling miserable. Peace of mind enters when you let go and allow the anxiety to manifest as it is without any resentment or resistance toward it. We forgive in order to heal and move on with our lives.

In a very gentle way, forgiveness peels away the layers of anxiety. As these layers fall, you start to uncover something new: a possibility that was hidden from you until you discovered the gift that was in disguise. This is the second stage in the perceptual switch:

2. DISCOVER MEANING

Sometimes things happen for a reason.

In his book *Traveling Light*, Daniel O'Leary writes, "As with anger, once we enlist and utilize the energy of fear in our favor, we move along our path to wholeness with swifter feet."

Could your whole journey through anxiety actually be one of the most valuable lessons in your life? Could anxiety be your greatest teacher?

I believe anxiety can enable you to grow and develop in ways that may not have been possible before. You see, once a person really faces their anxiety issue, they develop an inner strength that the average person never gets to develop. Real strength comes from facing a challenge like anxiety and learning to function all the while with it. You build that confidence each time you implement The DARE Response.

Existential philosopher Soren Kierkegaard was speaking to this idea when he wrote: *"Whoever has learned to be anxious in the right way has learned the ultimate."*

You really can find meaning in this suffering by determining your own response to anxiety. No longer thinking like a victim, you have freedom to take a stand—and that's nothing short of a triumph.

Despair is suffering without meaning. The simplest way to discover the meaning of your anxiety, the gift lurking beneath this unpleasant experience, is to write down the things you feel you're learning from your anxiety, and then write down the reason you want to succeed and overcome it.

For example:

-*What's the meaning of these panic attacks?*

Panic attacks are teaching me more about myself. This is a crash course in self-development.

-<u>Reason to overcome</u>:

I want to develop and become a bigger person.

-*What's the meaning of this constant anxiety?*

Anxiety is showing me where I hold myself back.

-<u>Reason to overcome</u>:

I want to live a more expansive, adventurous life.

-Why am I the only one who feels like this? What's the meaning of this?

Anxiety is teaching me greater compassion for others and myself.

-<u>Reason to overcome</u>:

I want to help others that are going through the same thing and teach them how to handle their anxiety and have courage.

Dr. Frankl says, "A human being, by the very attitude he chooses, is capable of finding and fulfilling meaning in even a hopeless situation." When you find meaning in your anxiety, you transcend it, and a new dimension of hope opens to you. Anytime you feel anxiety raise its head, remind yourself of the bigger picture and focus on that.

Only you can find the meaning to your personal challenge. Once you find that meaning, determine one or more reasons for overcoming that challenge. Your indomitable courage can become an inspiration to yourself and those that know you.

Remember the special journey you're on. Remember the gift anxiety holds for you. If you focus on this, you'll keep moving forward even on your most difficult of days.

Many never get to develop this inner strength of character that anxiety nurtures in us. When anxiety is overcome, you're left with an inner strength and confidence that you carry with you for the rest of your life.

The third and final practice involved in the perceptual switch of your anxiety is *gratitude.*

3. GRATITUDE

If you can reach the point where you're grateful for anxiety, you've made the full switch in perception that's needed to truly heal your anxiety. What a powerful place to come from. You look your tormentor in the eye and say thank you for being here.

It reminds me of someone I was coaching a while back. She said after so many years of anxiety and panic attacks, she could finally see the hidden gift of anxiety and was grateful for that. She developed a rock-solid sense of confidence that hadn't been there before.

"I see the anxiety as a messenger, an important tool to help me know myself. Working WITH my anxiety in this way is new for me, as I have suppressed my negative feelings for almost all of my adult life. When anxiety is hot in my chest and belly, I just say, 'Hello there, welcome, let's talk.' Then later in the day when I can relax, I come back to the feelings and accept their presence, thanking them for being around and the lessons they present me."

Just like forgiveness, gratitude is a force that lifts you above that which has been oppressing you.

Here is a short story from an unknown author to help illustrate this point:

A man found a cocoon of an emperor moth. He took it home so that he could watch the moth come out of the cocoon. On the day a small opening appeared, he sat and watched the moth for several hours as the moth struggled to force its body through that little hole.

Then it seemed to stop making any progress. It appeared as if it had gotten as far as it could and it could go no farther. It just seemed to be stuck.

Then the man, in his kindness, decided to help the moth, so he took a pair of scissors and snipped off the remaining bit of the cocoon. The moth then emerged easily. But it had a swollen body and small, shriveled wings.

The man continued to watch the moth because he expected that, at any moment, the wings would enlarge and expand to be able to support the body, which would contract in time. Neither happened! In fact, the little moth spent the rest of its life crawling around with a swollen body and shriveled wings. It was never able to fly.

What the man, in his kindness and haste did not understand, was that the restricting cocoon and the struggle required for the moth to get through the tiny opening, was the way of forcing fluid from the body of the moth into its wings so that it would be ready for flight once it achieved its freedom from the cocoon. Freedom and flight would come only after the struggle. By depriving the moth of a struggle, he deprived the moth of its health and its freedom.

This story illustrates the point that within each problem—no matter how intense-seeming—there really can be a hidden gift. Anxiety is a harsh teacher, but now that you're finally ready to graduate from the lesson anxiety teaches, maybe you can see the growth you've achieved.

Far from being a curse, anxiety can be your teacher. It can help you grow and develop as a wiser, stronger and more compassionate human. I know this can be hard to see when you're feeling so "broken" right now, but if you allow it time, your cracks can mend and you can feel whole again.

GIVE UP YOUR CRUTCHES

This is a short chapter, but it contains an important final challenge for you. You need to pass this challenge in order to reach full recovery. If you've suffered from anxiety for any significant length of time, you'll have developed one or more crutches. Crutches can be people you rely on or things you use to help you feel reassured and safe in anxious situations.

Some typical examples might be:

- Always having a safe person with you

- Never leaving home without your cell phone

- Always having a Xanax in your pocket

- Carrying a small bottle of alcohol around with you

- Messaging or calling people each time you feel anxious

- Having the same medical exams performed over and over again

Crutches are any external thing that you feel you need in order to feel safe. It's understandable how crutches develop as they offer a safety net of sorts. You think to yourself, "Well, if things get really bad, I'll always have X to rely upon." If you think about it, needing a crutch is a sign that you still do not fully trust that you're safe. Crutches are an indication that you're still resisting the experience of anxiety.

In the early stages of recovery, crutches are very helpful to get you up and walking toward your goal. If you broke your leg, you would need crutches to get you mobile and moving. After a certain point, you then need to discard the crutches in order to stand firmly on your own two legs.

Here is how Ian described the process of giving up his biggest crutch (his wife).

I feel I've made amazing progress since joining the program. I'm doing things I haven't attempted in years. Anxiety and panic do not have the same impact on me they used to have. In fact, I haven't had a full-on actual panic attack in a couple months now. There is still lots of ground to be covered, and I don't feel I'm out the woods yet, but now I mostly feel positive about the journey that I'm on. This afternoon I read a post in the "members" area about "crutches." This got me thinking, and I then had a good chat with my wife. I explained to her that the support she's giving me is now holding me back. I thanked her for always being there for me, for doing the things I feel I can't, for being my company when I have to drive past my comfort zone.

I explained to her that I know she does all these things because she thinks she's helping me and that I thought that too, but from now on she's to never allow me to use her as a "crutch" again—no matter what.

I love my wife with all my heart, and I have no idea how I would have got through these last six years without her, but it's time I remove my "crutch" and continue this journey alone now.

Of course, this chat with her has made me anxious. It's given me a lot of what ifs. … What if I'm not ready or I'm having a bad day or I'm not as far down the road to recovery as I think I am and I still need her …?

But I'm answering all these with a big fat "so what." I'm expecting my anxiety levels to go up again in the next few weeks and maybe even a return of panic attacks, but for me this is now the next step I need to take, and even if I change my mind, it's too late. I've had the chat and I've asked her, "<u>No matter what I say, this is now the way to help me</u>."

What Ian did was dramatic and took a lot of courage. Part of him recognized that his recovery had plateaued, and in order to get to the next level, he needed to take this leap and discard his crutch.

I'm not suggesting that you need to discard your crutches with the same gusto as Ian did, but at the very least try to start the process and wean yourself off your crutches in incremental stages.

For example, today you might decide to go for a drive alone instead of taking your safe person with you. Maybe you could leave your phone or Xanax at home when you go out for a walk. Or maybe you could decide to go shopping locally on your own.

Whatever it is that you're always doing with your crutch, start to plan ways to practice without it. Try to do one small thing each day without your crutch. It doesn't have to be a big thing; the important thing is to keep pushing out so that you're building your confidence up like a muscle.

I know that this can be very hard to do in the initial stages, especially if you've relied upon your crutch for many years, but you have to now dig deep and find the courage. You're well equipped for this challenge because you now have The DARE Response to replace your crutch. It will teach you to rely solely on yourself anytime you feel anxious.

It is, of course, possible to have a good level of recovery with a crutch still in place, but you'll never feel like you've made it all the way. There will be this niggle of anxiety that will keep pestering you, telling you that you're still vulnerable as you still rely upon your crutch to feel safe. That niggle will undermine your confidence in the long run, and that's why this final challenge is so important to take.

Commit to doing it right now. Create a workable plan to discard your crutches so that you can achieve a full recovery.

Walk bravely forward into each new day.

SUPERCHARGE YOUR RECOVERY

We're coming close to the end of our journey together. I've introduced you to what I believe is the most powerful tool you can be equipped with to end your anxiety, The DARE Response. That tool alone is all you need to break free from anxiety and get you back to living your life to the fullest again.

But we're not at the end of the journey just yet. ... I want to finish by giving you some additional tips and insights. This advice will not only help you speed up the recovery process, but it's also a great way to keep anxiety at bay after your recovery. I use the tips below to keep my own anxiety in check anytime I'm going through a stressful period.

Some people write whole books on what I share below, but I've condensed the information down to just the essential information that you need. Please try to implement as many of the following tips as possible. They will truly supercharge your recovery and ensure a lasting success.

HEAL WITH YOUR HEART

An old English proverb says, "Fear knocked on the door; love answered, and no one was there."

As you're more familiar now with The DARE Response, I want to delve deeper into it and share an insight with you that can really help spur on your recovery.

I've spoken about the importance of getting your anxious mind out of the way to really break the anxiety loop, but what's actually driving the healing when you take your anxious mind out of the way? If you look at the core qualities of The DARE Response, you'll find things like acceptance, allowance, compassion, playfulness, and kindness. These are the real qualities that heal anxiety, and they are in fact qualities of the heart.

In the end, you heal anxiety with your heart, not your head. It's the light and warmth of a compassionate heart that clears the dense fog of anxiety. Your mind can manage and control anxiety to some degree, but it doesn't have the transformational power to heal it. That power comes up from the heart. When your anxious mind is taken out of the way, it's your heart that allows peace of mind to be restored.

There's intelligence in your heart, and the voice of the wiser, more grounded you comes from the heart. Your anxious mind needs to be reassured by this voice. It's the voice of your real and authentic self. Practicing allowance and acceptance is really about creating a space for this wiser, more compassionate voice to come to the fore and to soothe your anxious mind.

Your heart sees the bigger picture, which allows you to see your pain in a new light. Your heart understands the purpose and meaning in this struggle and gives you the courage to connect with life again.

When you're very anxious, you end up trapped in your head all the time—the prison without walls. Your heart has the ability to throw that prison door open and set you free. The way it does so is through *compassionate acceptance*. "It's okay," your heart says to your anxious mind. "I've got this one. I accept and allow this anxious feeling. You don't have to hold on so tightly anymore." This soft, compassionate acceptance of the anxiety reassures the anxious mind that things are, in fact, alright. Your mind feels less pressure to try to control everything.

Most people aren't aware that in 1983, the heart was reclassified as a hormonal gland. The heart produces important hormones, several of which are responsible for reducing the stress response. One of those hormones is called atrial natriuretic factor (ANF), and its job is to reduce the release of stress hormones in your body.

Another hormone called oxytocin, commonly referred to as the "love" hormone, is also a powerful stress-relieving hormone released by the heart. When we hug or kiss a loved one, oxytocin levels go up. Moments of empathy and compassion stimulate the release of the hormone, which triggers your relaxation response.

By adopting an attitude of compassionate acceptance toward your anxiety, you trigger the secretion of these stress-reducing hormones. So when I talk about the healing properties of the heart, I mean it both metaphorically as well as physically.

LOVE HEALS FEAR.

It's a message that's been passed down through the ages. Unfortunately, the concept is too abstract for practical application to a problem like an anxiety disorder. The DARE Response is a practical application of that wisdom. It's a therapeutic approach with heartfelt compassion at its core.

The Max Planck Institute for Human Cognitive and Brain Sciences is a leading research institute on the neuroscientific effects of compassion and mindfulness, and they conducted a major study in Germany called the ReSource Project. The findings of this project confirmed what thousands of other studies have shown, which is that meditation and mindfulness do have significant stress-reducing effects on participants. What was most interesting in their findings, however, was that when participants were trained on compassion-based exercises, their stress levels dropped significantly lower compared with using just mindfulness alone. What their study showed is that feelings of compassion can dramatically reduce a person's stress levels.

In order to get the full stress-reducing benefits of compassion, we need to practice feeling more compassion toward ourselves. As I mentioned previously, we all tend to beat ourselves up way too much for having an anxiety problem. When you begin to adopt an approach like The DARE Response, you start a fundamental shift in the way you feel about yourself and your anxiety. Developing a compassionate acceptance of who you are and what you're experiencing is the key to reducing stress and improving your own self-image and self-worth.

Modern psychology is only now starting to grasp the transformative power of working with compassion in therapeutic practice. We're seeing a real growth of interest in therapies like mindfulness-based cognitive therapy (MBCT) and acceptance and commitment therapy (ACT), which are in reality heart-centered therapies. As mentioned previously, I predict these heart-centered therapeutic approaches will soar in popularity over the coming years as they outperform older therapeutic practices.

Your heart is the true healer. As you practice The DARE Response, you're not just working on reducing your anxiety in the best way possible, but you're also working on improving your sense of self-worth, which will supercharge your recovery!

WATER

The next tool I want you to use to supercharge your recovery is water. Water is a great quencher of thirst, but more importantly here, it's a great quencher of anxiety. There is no quicker way to significantly reduce general anxiety than drinking fresh water.

Nearly every function of the body is connected to the efficient flow of water through our system. Water transports hormones, chemical messengers, and nutrients to vital organs of the body. When we don't keep our bodies well hydrated, our bodies then start to react with a variety of signals, some of which are symptoms of anxiety. Studies have shown that being just half a liter (the equivalent of two cups) dehydrated can increase your cortisol levels, making you feel more anxious and on edge.

When you're suffering from frequent panic attacks, your stress response is firing more than usual, and this creates a buildup of toxins in your system that need to be flushed out. This is why it's so important to keep yourself well hydrated all the time.

The key to rebalancing a deficit of fluids is to drink eight glasses of fresh water daily. *However, you must spread this intake throughout the day and not drink it all in one go.* Otherwise, your body won't have a chance to absorb it, and the excess will just pass through your body. Sip your water throughout the day for maximum absorption. I would caution against drinking too much before bed, though, only because it might disrupt your sleep if you need to use the bathroom in the middle of the night.

The easiest way to ensure you're getting enough is to make it easy for yourself by having water placed in strategic locations. That might mean having fresh bottled water in the car, at your desk, or any place you know you spend time. If you place it in visible positions, you'll drink it. If it's out of sight, it quickly goes out of mind. With any new habit you want to form, you have to make it easy for yourself or else you'll drop it after a few days.

When you're aware that dehydration is a factor that contributes to anxiety and nervousness, you start to pay much greater attention to how much you're drinking daily. Personally, I've found that not only does a regular intake of water ward off any subtle feelings of anxiety, but it's also incredibly useful for building stamina and avoiding fatigue. Increasing the amount of fresh water you drink to eight glasses a day is a very easy step to incorporate into your daily routine, and it can have such a huge impact on your recovery from anxiety.

DIET

There are three things you must cut out of your diet if you want to truly speed your recovery process. Before I tell you what those are, it's worth mentioning that the ideal diet for anyone suffering from anxiety is a low glycemic diet.

That basically means a diet that keeps your blood sugar levels constant throughout the day. The reason for this is that symptoms of panic and anxiety can often be very similar to the symptoms of low blood sugar levels. If your blood sugar levels fluctuate too much, your body ends up releasing more adrenaline into your system, making you feel more on edge. In fact, a person's first panic attack can often be caused by a sudden drop in blood sugar levels— for example, after a night out of excessive drinking or eating, as we'll see below.

Because foods with a low glycemic index take longer to digest, they maintain blood sugar (glucose) levels at a relatively constant state throughout the day.

For the initial stages of recovery, however, I don't want you starting a new diet. Instead, I want you to focus just on cutting the worst offenders out of your current diet. That alone will be more than beneficial in speeding up your recovery.

Here are the things that absolutely must go in order for you to speed up your recovery:

ELIMINATE CAFFEINE

Caffeine is a powerful stimulant that can make you feel very nervous, anxious, and jittery. I'm constantly amazed by how many well-educated people come to me for help and have never made the connection between the amount of coffee they drink and the sensitization they feel.

Common bodily sensations caused by caffeine are fast heartbeat, irritability, headaches, and muscle tremors. For a sensitized person, these can be enough to trigger anxiety or even a panic attack.

The world seems to be in a love affair with coffee. I do enjoy it myself, but for people suffering from anxiety, it really has to go. The price you pay is too high. Besides coffee, caffeine is also found in energy drinks (avoid them at all cost), black tea, chocolate, and a number of weight-loss pills.

ALCOHOL

Next on the list of items that have to go is alcohol. Like coffee, our culture revolves around alcohol, especially in social situations. It can be nice to have a few drinks to help you relax, but the resulting hangover is just not worth it—especially if you suffer from anxiety or panic.

Hangovers result from dehydration and electrolyte imbalance. I'm sure many of you are familiar with the "the hangover fear." This is a heightened sense of anxiety and jumpiness that results from the dehydration of a hangover.

The surest way for someone who suffers from high anxiety to experience yet more anxiety is to drink excessive amounts of alcohol and wait for the hangover to set in the following day. I hear lots of stories of people having their first panic attack after a big party the night before. More often than not, all it takes is a little stress mixed with a bad hangover to trigger a full-blown panic attack.

It can be difficult to avoid alcohol completely, but you should at the very least stop drinking it until you're through your recovery phase and not feeling so sensitized to anxiety anymore.

AVOID EXCESS SUGAR

You know now that you want to avoid too much of a variation in your blood sugar levels so that there's less adrenaline released into your system throughout the day. The best way to do this is to cut out foods that are very high in sugar. That means sweets, cakes, chocolate, soft drinks, and ice cream should all be eliminated—at least until you're feeling much less anxious. I mentioned at the start I don't want you to change your diet too much as it's just not sustainable, but just cutting back on the really high sugar items will make a massive difference in how you feel.

SUPPLEMENTS

There's a ton of information—and most of it's misleading—about which supplements work best in reducing feelings of anxiety. The two supplements I recommend most often to people are **magnesium** and **calcium**.

Almost half the US population has an inadequate intake of magnesium in their diet due to not eating enough dark-green leafy vegetables and whole grains. Magnesium is the relaxation mineral and is essential for about 300 different biochemical reactions in the body. It relaxes the nervous system, enabling you to feel less sensitized. It promotes better sleep and helps maintain a healthy heart.

Dr. Mark Hynman goes so far as to say that if you're feeling tight, irritable, crampy, and stiff in your mind or body, it's a sign of magnesium deficiency. A recent scientific review of magnesium concluded, "It is highly regrettable that the deficiency of such an inexpensive, low-toxicity nutrient results in diseases that cause incalculable suffering and expense throughout the world."

Magnesium is often nicknamed "the original chill pill" because it acts on the regulation of the stress response by reducing the amount of stress hormones (e.g., cortisol and adrenaline) that are released at any one time.

But not all magnesium is equal, and how you take it is also a factor. It's key to bring to light that in order to get the best absorption of magnesium, you need to supplement it with calcium.

The reason for this is that calcium and magnesium are very similar minerals. They sit right next to each other on the periodic table and have the same two-plus charge. What that means is that if you're deficient in calcium, the enzymes that actually need calcium can't get it and start to rob the magnesium, even though it's not suited for them. This then reduces the amount of magnesium available in your body for the correct enzymes. So the advice now is to take both magnesium and calcium together to avoid this problem.

How much and when to take it?

To start, I recommend 250 mg of magnesium and 500 mg of calcium daily with your evening meal. After a week, you can then double that amount by taking the same dose at breakfast time as well.

One thing you have to know about magnesium is that it does cause increased bowel movements and loosened stool for most people. Don't be alarmed by that; it's very common. If diarrhea develops, however, stop taking the magnesium for a few days and then reintroduce it slowly again.

The type of magnesium and calcium you buy is important. For magnesium buy magnesium citrate, hydroxyapatite, or gluconate. Avoid magnesium carbonate, sulfate, aspartate, or oxide as they don't have the desired effect.

For calcium you can use calcium carbonate or citrate. They're the most popular supplement types. Others also exist, such as calcium gluconate and calcium phosphate. Avoid oyster shell, which is a form of calcium carbonate that's been known to occasionally contain small amounts of lead, a toxin.

Here's a final warning about taking these supplements: Since magnesium is excreted by the kidneys, people with heart or kidney disease as well as the elderly shouldn't take magnesium supplements except under their doctor's supervision. I always advise people who have concerns to speak to their doctor before taking any supplements.

For more information on supplements to reduce anxiety visit: www.dareresponse.com/audio

EXERCISE

The next area that will cause a massive reduction in your anxiety levels is exercise. You're likely very aware of how good exercise is for your body, but are you aware how good it is for your mind?

If you're looking for a magic pill to elevate your mood and reduce feelings of anxiety, exercise is the closest thing we currently have. Dopamine, serotonin, and norepinephrine are critical neurotransmitters that regulate your mood and behavior. So if you want a sudden boost in mood, you can have it for free anytime you want—all you have to do is exercise. In fact, Dr. Robert Butler once said that *if there was a drug that provided all the positive benefits of exercise, the whole world would be taking it!*

There are countless studies that prove how beneficial exercise is for our mood because it helps reduce feelings of anxiety and depression. Exercise is the best antidepressant we have (the best anxiety inhibitor). John Ratey, MD is a clinical professor of psychiatry at Harvard Medical School and one of the leading scientists on the science of exercise. In his book *Spark: The Revolutionary New Science of Exercise and the Brain*, he explains how exercise is as effective in reducing depression as taking the most commonly prescribed antidepressant, Zoloft.

Now think of all the extra health benefits you get from exercise that you don't get from taking a pill—and in addition, there are no side effects! What's even more amazing to consider is the negative impact *not* exercising has on our mental health.

Tal Ben Shahar says *not exercising is actually like taking a depressant!* People who don't exercise are much more prone to anxiety and depression. The reason is that exercising produces a protein called "brain-derived neurotrophic factor," or as Dr. Ratey calls it, "Miracle-Gro for the brain." According to Ratey, this protein encourages new neurons to grow and protects them from stress and cell death. Low levels of this protein have been associated with depression and even suicide. You can have this miracle protein in abundance for free, and all you have to do is exercise! So why are so few of us doing it?

The problem of course is motivation. Exercise takes commitment and effort. The less you exercise, the less you want to. The good news is that once you get over the initial hurdle, it starts to get a lot easier as more energy and motivation are available to you. Then the reverse happens—the more you exercise, the more you want to.

The very best way to motivate yourself to exercise in the beginning is to make it enjoyable. That means finding a way to exercise that you'll look forward to. For many this means a type of team sport or at least having a workout buddy, i.e., running with a friend or having a gym partner. In addition, exercising with another person makes you accountable so that it's harder to skip a session than if you're on your own. You can add to this the boost in mood from the social interaction.

How much do you need to exercise?

Researchers at the University of Texas Southwest Medical Center found a reduction of depressive symptoms after individuals exercised for thirty minutes three to five times per week over twelve weeks. High-intensity activity produced a 47 percent reduction, while low-intensity activity resulted in a 30 percent reduction.

A high-intensity activity is defined by your heart rate being elevated while you break a sweat. Examples might be strenuous walking, hiking, rowing, biking, running, or weight lifting. Talk to your doctor to make sure you know which activities, how much exercise, and what intensity level is right for you. Your doctor will consider any medications you take and health conditions you have.

I'm sure in years to come we'll look back and see that exercise was one of the most underutilized methods for maintaining good mental health.

LAUGHTER

Laughter is one of the best ways to snap a person out of an anxious state of mind. The problem is that as we get older, we have fewer opportunities to have a good laugh, which is a real shame if you consider just how beneficial it is for our health.

Data is mounting about the positive things laughter can do. Doctors even call laughing "inner jogging" because it induces positive changes in your body, such as the following:

- Levels of stress hormones such as cortisol decrease during bouts of laughter.

- It lowers blood pressure and increases vascular blood flow.

- It increases your tolerance for pain by releasing endorphins.

- It enhances your intake of oxygen-rich air and stimulates your heart, lungs, and muscles.

Robin Dunbar, a psychologist at Oxford, conducted several studies on the way laughter can increase resistance to pain. He demonstrated that laughter is only really powerful when the laughter is physical. What that means is that it's not enough to find something amusing (cerebral humor); you have to have a good physical laugh to trigger enough endorphins to get the feel-good effect.

You also need to laugh with others for the best effect. As with choosing a workout partner, you get the benefit of social connections in addition to the intrinsic value of laughter.

The interesting thing about laughing is that, just like yawning, it's contagious. You don't even have to know what you're laughing about in order to start. You just have to give yourself permission to do so.

In my opinion one of the best places for you to be spending your free time if you suffer from anxiety or panic is at a stand-up comedy gig. This works well because just being in a room full of people who are laughing has a contagious effect. It doesn't matter if you don't even find the comics that funny. Just go there with the explicit intention of laughing. What you'll find is that if you go in with that attitude, then when everyone else starts laughing, you'll just go along with it.

I'm a huge advocate of using laughter to boost mood and reduce anxious feelings. I know many people who have transformed their anxiety by doing just this one thing alone! Think of your comedy nights out as essential therapy, not merely as entertainment. Make it a date night with your partner or a chance to socialize with friends.

If a comedy show isn't a possibility for you, then the next best thing is to have friends around who you know will make you laugh and either play a party game together (e.g., charades) or watch a funny movie.

Most people will overlook this tip of using laughter, or they'll consider it frivolous, but I urge you to at least try it and notice how you feel the following day. Again, it's one of those simple tips that's easy to implement and incredibly enjoyable to do. Don't let the small effort it takes to make it happen stop you from potentially feeling so much better.

GUIDED RELAXATION

A daily practice of listening to a guided relaxation is the final tip I want to share to help you supercharge your recovery from anxiety. It's very important to practice this daily, especially if you're the kind of person who experiences anxiety each day on waking. Guided relaxation works by enabling you to consciously produce the body's natural relaxation response, characterized by slower breathing, lower blood pressure, and a feeling of calm and well-being.

Being able to produce the relaxation response using relaxation techniques not only reduces feelings of anxiety, but it can also be very beneficial for aiding digestive disorders, headaches, high blood pressure, and insomnia.

Instead of just talking about it, though, I want you to experience it for yourself. I have a guided relaxation audio that I share with everyone I coach. People report a dramatic reduction in their anxiety levels when they use it daily over a period of three weeks. The audio I created, called "deep release," is designed specifically for people who suffer from high anxiety. To access the audio visit

www.DareResponse.com/app

I recommend you listen to it at least once a day, ideally in the morning or before bed at night. Listening to the audio daily is an incredibly effective way to improve your all-around sense of well-being.

KEEP PUSHING OUT

To really progress fast you need to always be pushing out through your anxiety. Each day think of at least one thing that you can do to push outside your safe zone. Plan out what you're going to do the night before and then get up and go for it.

It's too easy to read a book like this and then not take consistent action. Please take action, and please stick with it. I know you have what it takes, so don't give up on yourself, even when you're in a deep rut.

Keep getting up, keep pushing out, keep demanding more. *That's the very fastest way to get your life back.*

HANDING OVER TO A HIGHER POWER

Finally for those of you who believe in God regardless of your faith, it is important to highlight the great strength and peace of mind that can be drawn from spiritual practise. Almost all religions and spiritual beliefs talk about the importance of surrendering your fears and worries over to God when you are feeling anxious. You are advised to surrender your concerns over to that higher power and trust that you will be looked after. This intention or prayer not only quietens an anxious mind but it also helps reduce the isolation felt when fearful.

The final step in the Dare response (engage) is a great opportunity to do this. As you engage back with life again you can pray that God (or whatever higher power you believe in) will look after you. You surrender over to that power and trust that your anxiety issue will be resolved. You are not pushing the anxiety away instead it is a belief you hold that something more powerful than you is now looking after this issue for you and that you need not spend any more of your time worrying or obsessing over it. You engage with life fully trusting that you are cared for and looked after.

NOW DO IT!

I want to point out that you can of course just use The DARE Response to heal your anxiety (and many people do), but why not give yourself as much support along the way as possible and speed your recovery by implementing the additional tools I've outlined in this chapter? If you find it too challenging to implement them all, then choose the ones that resonate the most with you and start them today. I would prefer you did one or two of them well rather than trying to do them all only halfheartedly.

CONCLUSION

> No one saves us but ourselves. No one can and no one may. We ourselves must walk the path.
>
> – Buddha

The whole purpose of this book and The DARE Response is for you to win back your freedom—to get you living life again without the shadow of anxiety hanging over you. I know that's what you long for the most: To live without having to think each situation through in advance. To be able to go places without the fear of what might happen when you get there. To spend time with friends or family without the constant intrusion of anxious thoughts.

Life is movement. The DARE Response is the way to move you back into life again. It's no coincidence that the last step of The DARE Response is "engage." That step completes the circle and moves you back into the life that anxiety stole from you. You can see how this movement into life acts in opposition to anxiety. Anxiety takes you out of life. The DARE Response places you right back in it.

Every time you practice The DARE Response, you're aiding the recovery process and healing your anxiety. That's why I say you can never fail at applying The DARE Response, even if your anxiety doesn't drop immediately. Just the very act of implementing it is something to celebrate as it always gets you moving in the right direction. Don't doubt yourself or the process. Simply trust that it's working, and over a short period of time, you'll start to feel a whole lot better. You have to keep doing this brave work. Remember, you're the cure. No one else can do it for you.

Do you remember at the start of the book I dared you to imagine what your life might look like without anxiety being an issue anymore? Well, you now have *the tools* to absolutely achieve that. I hope you're starting to feel a lot more hopeful about your future. I hope that the dreams you may have been putting on hold are starting to come alive once more and are exciting you.

When you commit to and continuously practice The DARE Response, you quickly start to feel more comfortable in your own skin again. You feel more engaged with life and less worried about situations that troubled you before. Deep down you start to finally trust that no matter what happens, you can bravely handle it.

Remember, *recovery is not the absence of sensations.* It's about living life regardless of what sensations are present and not letting those sensations get in the way of what you want to do. Eventually over time those sensations fall away all by themselves because you no longer pay them any heed.

The only way out is through. Of course, there will be setbacks along the way, but as long as you understand that these setbacks are a key part of the recovery process, they won't hinder you.

In the beginning no one feels like they're making progress fast enough, but trust me: if you're doing the work, you're healing at the right speed for you. Through complete acceptance and nonresistance of your anxious sensations, you'll eventually set yourself free.

Very soon, one of these mornings, you'll wake and feel like a layer of anxiety has fallen away from your life. Then, a few weeks later, another layer will fall away, and then another, and another. Eventually you'll be back to your old self, but it's not quite the same old you. It's a new, more confident you that comes about through the mastery of your anxiety.

Time is your most precious resource. Don't waste any more of it on anxiety. Life is waiting for you—go out and join it! I dare you to. You've been away too long.

Barry McDonagh

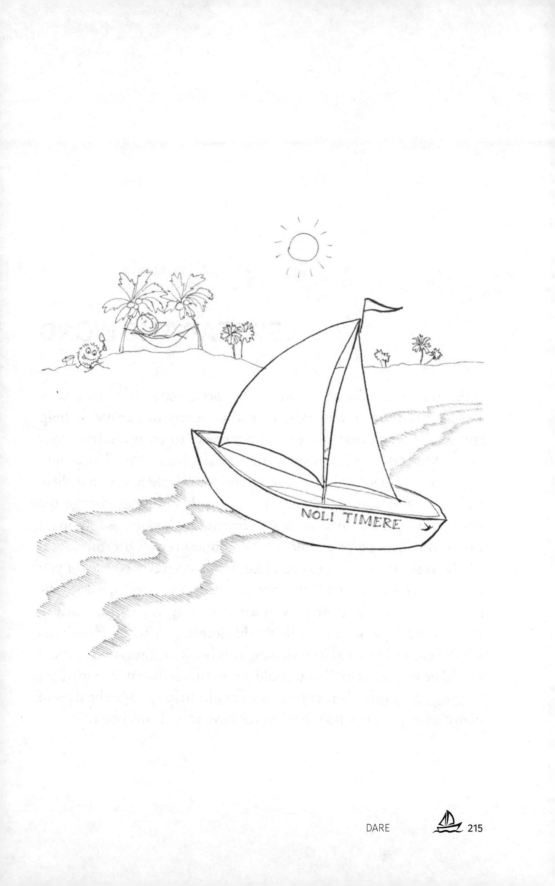

SPREAD THE WORD

If this book has helped you, *please help spread the word. Send a tweet or post something on Facebook.* **I need an army of people to help spread the word that there is a better way to treat anxiety.** Your message could help reach someone who's suffering in silence right now. Together we can shine a light and let people know that there really is a solution to this problem. Together we can change the current culture of 'anxiety management' to 'anxiety solution'. I would also love it if you could leave an honest review on Amazon. It can be as short or as long as you like. Write whatever is true for you and your experience with this book. Your review will speak to the people who experience anxiety in the same way as you do. Lastly, if you know people in the media world (journalists/bloggers/writers) who might be intrested in reviewing this book or interviewing me, I would be very grateful if you could get in touch by email at media@dareresponse.com. Your connections could help change the lives of many more people who would never have found this book.

COACHING

Sometimes people need live support to really help them move to a full recovery quicker. If you want that then join my coaching program, which runs every month. The coaching program is the very best way to get specific guidance and support from people who understand exactly what you're going through. The insight and help you'll get can really help you achieve your goals with greater ease. To learn more about that, visit: www.DareResponse.com/Coaching

STAY IN TOUCH!

Please let me know how you get on. I really do want to hear from you. You can message me directly on Facebook here.

www.facebook.com/BarryJoeMcDonagh

APPENDIX

Empirical Evidence for The DARE Response written by Dr. Joan Swart, PsyD

The DARE Response approach is aligned with a group of modern cognitive therapy approaches, commonly referred to as the third wave of therapies. These were derived from basic principles of cognitive theory, but distinguished in important perspectives.

The fathers of cognitive theory Drs. Aaron Beck (1964a; 1964b) and Albert Ellis (1957; 1962), as well as those who followed them, realized in the 1960s how important thoughts are to our wellbeing and behavior. Often negative thoughts arise automatically and result in unpleasant feelings and emotions. We also tend to compensate or deal with these distresses by acting in irrational and unhelpful ways. When we have instinctive thoughts of fear or threat our emotions and bodies react with panic and anxiety. These feelings are designed to make us act to avoid or eliminate the perceived threat. But the problem often is that our perceptions are misguided and lack sound reasoning. Beck (1964b) described such distorted thinking as reflecting "typical chronic misconceptions, distorted attitudes, invalid premises, and unrealistic goals and expectations" (p. 563). Similarly, Ellis (1957) argued that "what we call emotion is nothing more than a certain kind—a biased, prejudiced kind—of thought, and that human beings can be taught to control their feelings by controlling their thoughts." (p. 344).

With this simple understanding of how thoughts, feelings, and behavior relate, Cognitive Behavioral Therapy, or CBT, was developed. When a person encounters a significant event, it is instinctively interpreted and meaning attached according to their personal set of values or beliefs. Core beliefs and schemas—complex clusters of beliefs—develop through life based on the sum total of our previous life experiences. It gives direction to our perception and how we view ourselves, others, and the world in general, whether we are inclined to have—or don't have—hope, trust, empathy, self-confidence, feelings of safety, etc. Described as "fundamental, inflexible, absolute, and generalized" (Rathod, Kingdon, Pinninti, Turkington, & Phiri, 2015, p. 17), core beliefs are essentially the lens through which we interpret our world and what happens to us. Negative core beliefs lead to negative thoughts when activated, which are often unhelpful as it causes unpleasant feelings and dysfunctional behavior (see Figure 1).

Based on these premises of cognitive theory, the main objective of the CBT approach is to change emotions and behavior by identifying and challenging (also called "disputing") automatic negative thoughts. The process is based on the concepts of experiential avoidance and cognitive fusion.

Experiential avoidance is our spontaneous tendency to avoid negative experiences. Our bodies and minds will instinctively do anything to avoid feeling bad, including getting panic attacks, lashing out in anger, and withdrawing into ourselves. In fact, experts argue that experiential avoidance is at the core of all our psychological problems and our inability to experience pleasure (Hayes, Wilson, Gifford, Follette, & Strosahl, 1996). It is said that virtually every psychological problem "begins [and is sustained] as an attempt to avoid or get rid of unwanted thoughts and feelings such as boredom, loneliness, anxiety, depression, and so on." (Harris, 2006, p. 4). Therefore cognitive therapies utilize concepts of cognitive defusion, reappraisal, and redirection and emotion regulation to improve thinking processes.

Figure 1: *Cognitive Behavioral Sequence*

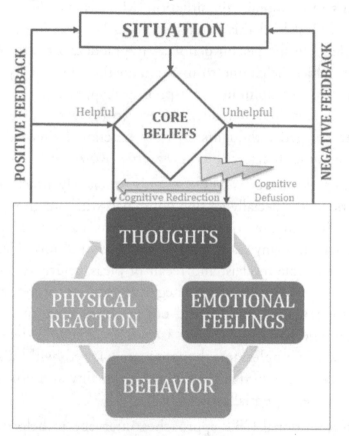

Emotion regulation refers to a person's ability to initiate, inhibit, or modulate emotional states in a given situation. But, rather than suppressing or avoiding undesirable feelings, which can lead to an even more distressed state, cognitive science has demonstrated that a redirection of attention or thoughts to healthier alternatives is more effective to improve self-regulation, mental state, and functional behavior (Goldin & Gross, 2010). *Cognitive reappraisal* is a particular adaptive type of emotion regulation, which was found to moderate the link between stress and anxiety symptoms (Ascher & Schotte, 1999). Instead of fighting one's fears—which typically increases the severity of symptoms—a reversal of the attitude away from avoidance enables the person to distance him- or herself from their fears and reappraise the situation (Michelson & Ascher, 1984). On a technical level this is referred to as *"paradoxical intention"*. In simpler terms, a person deliberately practices a fearful habit or thought, which helps one to understand the irrationality of their reaction. This is helpful in reinterpreting/reappraising the meaning of the activating event to reduce the severity of the negative response or redirect negative thoughts to more functional alternatives. The latter is commonly referred to as *cognitive redirection*.

Cognitive fusion happens where we subconsciously attach thoughts to experiences, especially getting entangled with our thoughts and allowing them to move or even overwhelm us. Cognitive fusion can be beneficial in many ways, such as attachment to love, identifying with positive role models, and recall of pleasant events. However, when thoughts are routinely negative we are prevented from pleasant experiences and instead engage in rumination (excessive worrying) and harmful behavior. *Cognitive defusion* is the opposite process where unpleasant thoughts are viewed with dispassion and unattachment so that they lose their quality and hold on self-identity and experiential avoidance.

As such, traditional CBT approaches intervene to help us defuse our negative thoughts from unpleasant experiences. While this is a positive goal, our thoughts and beliefs are discounted as unrealistic and irrational. Many find that such an approach has the opposite of the desired effect. Instead of being flawed, our negative thoughts are often based on an honest appraisal of how we interpret our reality. As such, it contains a "grain of truth" (Swart, Winters, &

Apsche, 2014, p. 7). Therefore, it is reasonable under our particular circumstances, although not always helpful or the best course of action.

Many researchers and practitioners found that a sizeable proportion of clients did not respond to CBT treatment, which they contributed to the fact that CBT lack focus on appraisal and acceptance (David & Szentagotai, 2006). It is because, in CBT, dysfunctional thoughts, feelings, and behavior are disputed as "bad" and attempts are made to change their contents or deny their existence altogether, which are often viewed as confrontational and invalidating. As a result, some clients find it difficult to stay positive and motivated. Eventually many abandon efforts to improve and grow.

Recognizing these shortcomings in the traditional CBT approach, experts added and adjusted selected core elements to improve the effectiveness of the cognitive-based change process. Mostly, **acceptance and validation replaced the attitude of disputation**. Linehan (1993) described validation in a psychology context as requiring the person to search for, recognize, and reflect the validity in response to events. According to Linehan, acceptance is an active process of tolerant embracing of how and who one is here and now, juxtaposed with acknowledging the necessity for change and growth. Furthermore, acceptance and validation is associated with the ability to find and express self-compassion and compassion for others, a feature that strongly counters the presence of depression and anxiety (Werner et al., 2012).

The concept of mindfulness was also added to standard CBT protocols to enhance focus on the present moment. Two common definitions of mindfulness are:

"[Mindfulness is] A kind of nonelaborative, nonjudgmental, present-centered awareness in which each thought, feeling, or sensation that arises in the attentional field is acknowledged and accepted as it is" (Bishop, et al., 2004, p. 282).

"Mindfulness means paying attention in a particular way, on purpose, in the present moment, and non-judgmentally" (Kabat-Zinn, 1994, p. 4).

This focused attention keeps the mind busy, thereby preventing us from constant worrying and self-identification with unpleasant thoughts and feelings. The attitude of acceptance and validation eliminates the need of avoidance. It also helps us understand that unpleasant experiences are a normal part of being, and do not define our worth. Neither is it permanent as our thoughts and feelings come and go constantly.

The major pillars of the new approach to negative thoughts are: "non-judging, patience, a beginner's mind, trust, non-striving acceptance, seeing things as they are in the present and letting go. They are all interconnected." (De Silva, 1979, p. 129). These elements all feature in the new therapies, which is a heterogeneous group of treatments, usually understood to include Acceptance and Commitment Therapy (DBT), Dialectical Behavior Therapy (DBT), Mindfulness-Based Cognitive Therapy (MBCT), Mode Deactivation Therapy (MDT), and Schema Therapy. The DARE Response as taught in this book is most consistent with the principles of ACT, DBT, and MDT.

Mode Deactivation Therapy (MDT) was originally developed to treat adolescents with severe conduct and personality disorders. Mindfulness, validation, and cognitive redirection are the central elements used to affect positive change in a systematic and goal-directed process. Appreciating the value in exploring the origins of maladaptive thought processes in past experiences, MDT also has a psychoanalytical, or past-oriented, component, which standard CBT does not employ.

Dialectical Behavior Therapy (DBT) is a cognitive behavioral treatment that was originally developed to treat chronically suicidal and borderline personality disorder patients. DBT combines strategies of behavior therapy and mindfulness practices with activities to enhance dialectical thinking patterns—the ability to synthesize opposite views—to replace rigid, dichotomous thinking (Dimeff & Linehan, 2001). Validation and acceptance are core elements in DBT.

Acceptance and Commitment Therapy (ACT) is a psychological intervention that also utilizes "acceptance and mindfulness strategies, together with commitment and behavior change strategies, to increase psychological flexibility." (Curren, 2009, p. 210). The approach emphasizes values, forgiveness, compassion, living in the present moment, and accessing a transcendent sense of self, instead of a primary objective to reduce symptoms (Harris, 2006). Psychological flexibility is defined as the capacity of a person to (1) adapt to fluctuating situational demands, (2) reconfigure mental resources, (3) shift perspective, and (4) balance competing desires, needs, and life domains (Kashdan & Rottenberg, 2010).

A plethora of research studies, including meta-analyses, concluded that the new approach is indeed more effective, or at least as effective, as traditional Cognitive Behavioral Therapy across a broad range of psychological problems. A meta-analysis is a statistical method for combining results from different studies in order to strengthen conclusions and highlight patterns. Selected third wave therapies were found to perform as follows:

A meta-analysis study by Ruiz (2012) that included a combined 954 participants found that ACT was effective and outperformed CBT to some degree in 11 of the 16 studies that were included. ACT especially led to better post-treatment quality-of-life outcomes, while also reducing symptoms of depression and anxiety.

Analyzing an overall number of 699 adolescents with behavioral and other problems, including depression and anxiety, Swart and Apsche (2014) found that MDT performed better than standard CBT and treatment-as-usual protocols. On average problematic behavioral symptoms were reduced by more than 30%.

DBT was found to halve the typical rate of suicide attempts among depressed patients, and patients were three times less likely to drop out of treatment compared to non-specific community and outpatient treatments (Linehan et al., 2006). DBT patients also improved significantly more than participants on waiting list controls on variables including depression, anxiety, interpersonal functioning, social adjustment, global psychopathology and self-injury (Bohus et al., 2004).

As a whole, there are not yet enough well-controlled studies to conclude that third wave therapies are conclusively more effective than other active treatments across a range of problems, including anxiety, but so far the data seem promising. This suggests that the mindfulness- and acceptance-based approaches are viable, possibly with longer-term and more stable improvement outcomes, and affect change in a distinctly person-centered way (Forman, Herbert, Moitra, Yeomans, & Geller, 2007). The third wave therapies' conceptualization of cognition—how thoughts interact with situations, beliefs, and emotions—rests on awareness and acceptance in order to distance oneself from negative thoughts. In technical terms this is also known as cognitive defusion and redirection.

In the proprietary Right Move process the acceptance, cognitive defusion, reappraisal, and redirection steps are framed as *Defuse*, *Allow*, *Get Excited/Demand More* and *Engage*. The DARE Response's **Defuse** step is about awareness of the trigger and instinctive reaction to anxiety. Such awareness eliminates worry and "what if?" thoughts, which quickly escalates situations that are perceived as threatening by causing distressed emotions, bodily sensations, and unhelpful behavior. External feedback that results from such behavior is usually poor, which further exacerbates the situation, including interpersonal interactions. Instead, the person is taught to accept his/her experiences as natural and passing, which defuses the intense thoughts and feelings. **The cognitive arousal is not resisted, but simply accepted. It is allowed to be, and, eventually,**

to pass. This step in The DARE Response method is similar to *mindfulness and awareness* in third wave therapies.

The second Right Move step is to **Allow** anxiety to exist, not to avoid it, but to move with it. Thereby, the irresistible impulse to do anything to avoid unpleasant experiences is removed. Essentially, our thoughts are distanced from our usual perceptions and the meanings that we attach to events. **By loosening our thoughts from our experiences, its hold on our self-identity weakens, we are enabled to regulate our emotions better**. The second step in The DARE Response method relates to *cognitive defusion* in third wave therapy approaches.

The third Right Move step in the management of severe anxiety and panic attacks is **Get Excited/Demand More**. Anxiety is purely a wave of energy that is not harmful by itself, unless interpreted as such and transformed into a growing negative force. Instead Right Move proposes to accept and utilize the energy—similar to the psychological concept of paradoxical intention. By changing our perception and interpretation of the stimulus, our perspectives become more positive and helpful. As soon as we are able to **reappraise our feelings of anxiety as something positive such as excitement, the situation becomes an opportunity rather than a threat and functioning/performance typically improves** (Brooks, 2014). Therefore, the third step in The DARE Response method follows the psychological principles of *paradoxical intention* and *cognitive reappraisal*.

The fourth Right Move step is to **Engage** your mind in a focused activity. This prevents a person's Default Mode Network (DMN) from activating. In neuroscience, the DMN is a network of brain regions that are active when the individual is not focused on the outside world and the brain is at wakeful rest. An increase in DMN activity is associated with rumination, resulting in higher levels of depression and anxiety (Nolen-Hoeksema, 2000). **Engaging in nonself-referential goal-directed tasks reduces DMN activity, in**

effect redirecting the mind away from worry. The fourth step in The DARE Response method is similar to *cognitive redirection* in third wave therapy approaches.

Table 1: *Change Mechanisms*

Step	Right Move	The Tool	Objectives
1	Defuse	Mindful awareness	Awareness of automatic thoughts
2	Allow	Acceptance; Cognitive defusion	Allow unpleasant experiences to exist through cognitive defusion.
3	Get excited, Demand more	Cognitive reappraisal; Paradoxical intention	Allow the symptoms, but reinterpret the meaning of the stimulus
4	Engage	Cognitive redirection	Reduce DMN activity and redirect attention and thought contents to focused goal-directed tasks

There are more similarities between The DARE Response and basic third wave therapy approaches than the primary steps and their objectives summarized in Figure 1. Both are based on basic cognitive theory and the principles of mindfulness, acceptance, and validation to reduce the meaning of negative thoughts. Thereby the negative thoughts - feelings - behavior chain reaction is disrupted to eliminate or redirect unhelpful thinking.

Therefore, it is evident that The DARE Response method is procedurally and theoretically sound as it is based on widely accepted and proven principles of cognitive science. The procedures and steps are well-defined and consistent with evidence-based third wave psychotherapy approaches. The methodology is framed in the familiar third wave psychotherapy principles of mindfulness, cognitive defusion, reappraisal, and redirection (see Figure 2), but at an accessible and user-friendly level that is also normalizing and validating.

Figure 2: *Cognitive Model of Third Wave Therapies*

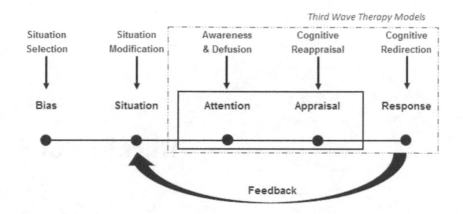

Compared to the basic cognitive model of third wave therapies that are based on the emotion regulation model of Stanford Professor James Gross and illustrated in Figure 1 (Gross & Barrett, 2012), The DARE Response approach is equally systematic and structured and utilizes clearly defined goals to motivate and direct users.

REFERENCES

Ascher, L. M., & Schotte, D. E. (1999). Paradoxical intention and recursive anxiety. *Journal of Behavior Therapy and Experimental Psychiatry, 30*(2), 71-79. DOI: 10.1016/S0005-7916(99)00009-9

Beck, A. T. (1964a). Thinking and depression: Idiosyncratic content and cognitive distortions. *Archives of General Psychiatry, 9*(4), 324-333. DOI: 10.1001/archpsyc.1964.01720160014002

Beck, A. T. (1964b). Thinking and depression: Theory and practice. *Archives of General Psychiatry, 10*(6), 561-571. DOI: 10.1001/archpsyc.1964.01720240015003

Bishop, S. R., Lau, M., Shapiro, S., Carlson, L., Anderson, N. D., Carmody, J.,...Devins, G. (2004). Mindfulness: A proposed operational definition. *Clinical Psychology: Science and Practice, 11*(3), 230-241. DOI: 10.1093/clipsy/bph077

Bohus, M., Haaf, B., Simms, T., Limberger, M. F., Schmal, C., Unckel, C.,...Linehan, M. M. (2004). Effectiveness of inpatient dialectical behavioral therapy for borderline personality disorder: A controlled trial. *Behavior Research and Therapy, 42*(5), 487-499. DOI: 10.1016/S0005-7967(03)00174-8

Brooks, A. W. (2014). Get excited: Reappraising pre-performance anxiety as excitement. *Journal of Experimental Psychology: General, 143*(3), 1144-1158. DOI: 10.1016/S0005-7916(99)00009-9

Curren, L. (2009). Trauma competency: A clinician's guide. Eau Claire, WI: PESI.

David, D., & Szentagotai, A. (2006). Cognitions in cognitive-behavioral psychotherapies; toward an integrated model. *Clinical Psychology Review, 26*(3), 284-298. DOI: 10.1016/j.cpr.2005.09.003

De Silva, P. (1979). *An introduction to Buddhist psychology.* New York, NY: Barnes & Noble Books.

Dimeff, L., & Linehan, M. M. (2001). Dialectical behavior therapy in a nutshell. *The California Psychologist, 34*, 10-13.

Ellis, A. (1957). Outcome of employing three techniques of psychotherapy. *Journal of Clinical Psychology*, 13, 344–350.

Ellis, A. (1962). *Reason and emotion in psychotherapy.* Secaucus, NJ: Citadel.

Forman, E. M., Herbert, J. D., Moitra, E., Yeomans, P. D., & Geller, P. A. (2007). A randomized controlled effectiveness trial of Acceptance and Commitment Therapy and Cognitive Therapy for anxiety and depression. *Behavior Modification, 31*(6), 772-799. DOI: 10.1177/0145445507302202

Goldin, P. R., & Gross, J. J. (2010). Effects of Mindfulness-Based Stress Reduction (MBSR) on emotion regulation in social anxiety disorder. *Emotion, 10*(1), 83-91. DOI: 10.1037/a0018441

Gross, J. J., & Barrett, L. F. (2011). Emotion generation and emotion regulation: One or two depends on your point of view. *Emotion Review, 3*(1), 8-16. DOI: 10.1177/1754073910380974

Harris, R. (2006). Embracing your demons: An overview of Acceptance and Commitment Therapy. *Psychotherapy in Australia, 12*(4), 2-8.

Hayes, S. C., Wilson, K. G., Gifford, E. V., Follette, V. M., & Strosahl, K. (1996). Experiential avoidance and behavioral disorders: A functional dimensional approach to diagnosis and treatment. *Journal of Consulting and Clinical Psychology, 64*(6), 1152-1168.

Kabat-Zinn, J. (1994). *Wherever you go there you are.* New York, NY: Hyperion.

Kashdan, T. B., & Rottenberg, J. (2010). Psychological flexibility as a fundamental aspect of health. *Clinical Psychology Review, 30*(7), 865-878. DOI: 10.1016/j.cpr.2010.03.001

Linehan, M. M. (1993). *Cognitive behavioral therapy of borderline personality disorder.* New York, NY: Guilford Press.

Linehan, M. M., Comtois, K. A., Murray, A. M., Brown, M. Z., Gallop, R. J., Heard, H. L.,…Lindenboim, N. (2006). Two-year randomized controlled trial and follow-up of Dialectical Behavior Therapy versus therapy by experts for suicidal behaviors and Borderline Personality Disorder. *Archives of General Psychiatry, 63*(7), 757-766. DOI: 10.1001/archpsyc.63.7.757

Michelson, L., & Ascher, L. M. (1984). Paradoxical intention in the treatment of agoraphobia and other anxiety disorders. *Journal of Behavior Therapy and Experimental Psychiatry, 15*(3), 215-220.

Nolen-Hoeksema, S. (2000). The role of rumination in depressive disorders and mixed anxiety/depressive symptoms. *Journal of Abnormal Psychiatry, 109*(3), 504-511. DOI: 101037/10021-843X.109.3.504

Rathod, S., Kingdon, D., Pinninti, N., Turkington, D., & Phiri, P. (2015). *Cultural adaptation of CBT for serious mental illness: A guide for training and practice.* Malden, MA: John Wiley & Sons.

Ruiz, F. J. (2012). Acceptance and Commitment Therapy versus traditional Cognitive Behavioral Therapy: A systematic review and meta-analysis of current empirical evidence. *International Journal of Psychology & Psychological Therapy, 12*(2), 333-357.

Swart, J., Winters, D., & Apsche, J. A. (2014). Mindfulness-based Mode Deactivation Therapy for adolescents with behavioral problems and complex comorbidity: Concepts in a nutshell and cost-benefit analysis. *Journal of Psychology & Clinical Psychiatry, 1*(5), 1-12. DOI: 10.15406/jpcpy.2014.01.00031

Swart, J., & Apsche, J. A. (2014). Mode deactivation therapy meta-analysis: Reanalysis and interpretation. *The International Journal of Behavioral Consultation and Therapy, 9*(2), 16-21.

Werner, K. H., Jazaieri, H., Goldin, P. R., Ziv, M., Heimberg, R. G., & Gross, J. J. (2012). Self-compassion and social anxiety disorder. *Anxiety, Stress, & Coping, 25*(5), 543-558. DOI: 10.1080/10615806.2011.608842

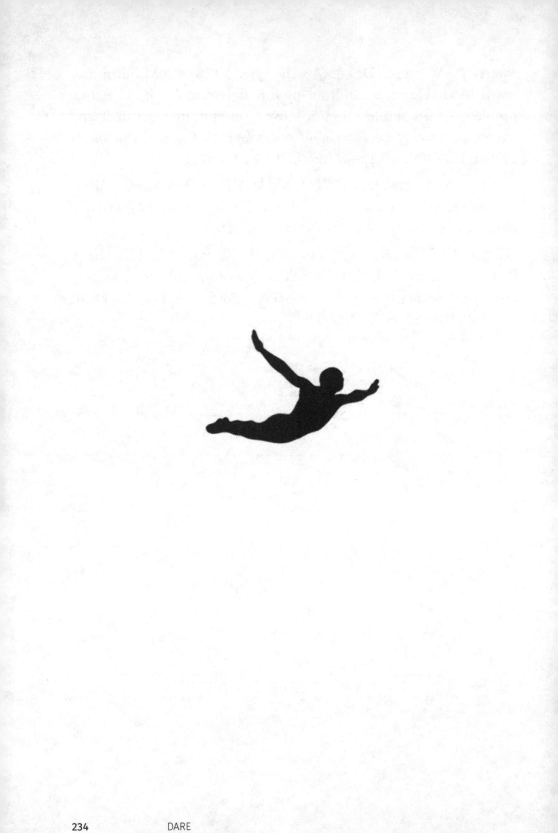

DARE

CPSIA information can be obtained
at www.ICGtesting.com
Printed in the USA
LVHW08s1547030918
589013LV00016B/666/P

9 780956 596253